NOTHING BUT THE TOOTH

NOTHING BUT THE TOOTH

An Insider's Guide to Dental Health

Teresa Yang, DDS

ROWMAN & LITTLEFIELD
Lanham • Boulder • New York • London

Published by Rowman & Littlefield
An imprint of The Rowman & Littlefield Publishing Group, Inc.
4501 Forbes Boulevard, Suite 200, Lanham, Maryland 20706
www.rowman.com

86-90 Paul Street, London EC2A 4NE

British Library Cataloguing in Publication Information Available

Library of Congress Cataloging-in-Publication Data

Names: Yang, Teresa (Dentist), author.
Title: Nothing but the tooth : an insider's guide to dental health / Teresa Yang, DDS.
Description: Lanham : Rowman & Littlefield, [2023] | Includes bibliographical references and index. | Summary: "A lively and approachable guide to all aspects of dental health"— Provided by publisher.
Identifiers: LCCN 2022056482 (print) | LCCN 2022056483 (ebook) | ISBN 9781538173657 (print) | ISBN 9781538173664 (ebook)
Subjects: LCSH: Teeth—Care and hygiene—Popular works.
Classification: LCC RK61 .Y36 2023 (print) | LCC RK61 (ebook) | DDC 617.6—dc23/eng/20230419
LC record available at https://lccn.loc.gov/2022056482
LC ebook record available at https://lccn.loc.gov/2022056483

CONTENTS

INTRODUCTION

I began writing this book, in my spare time, about ten years ago. As a practicing dentist for more than thirty years, I spent every day providing information to patients, answering their questions, and guiding them to better dental and overall health. It struck me that there was no single place for patients to gather information. Sure, they could ask Google a specific question. But what if they didn't even know what questions to ask?

Some of the topics I wanted to include in this book deal with areas for which Google may not have an answer, such as, "How do I find a good dentist?" or "Why is my dentist recommending this procedure when I don't have any sensitivity or symptoms?" or "Why is the implant advertised online so much cheaper than what my dentist quoted me?" I also wanted to talk about the mouth as an entry point to the body, that your dentist can spot a patient who suffers from bulimia, provide nutrition and oral care guidelines for people undergoing chemotherapy, or screen for sleep apnea.

I started to create an outline for the book and showed it to several of my colleagues. One called the project "ambitious" and said she was looking forward to retirement and playing tennis.

This got me thinking that maybe what I wanted to do *was* too ambitious. Why would I devote time and energy to writing a book about dentistry when no one really wanted to *go* to the dentist, much less read about it? I put the project on the back burner.

Fast-forward to 2021. For several months during the COVID-19 pandemic, I participated in mass vaccination efforts, preparing and delivering vaccines. When my coworkers—mostly nurses, medical assistants, and others from all walks of life—found out I was a dentist, they started speaking about their own dental experiences. They asked questions timidly at first, but soon the questions started coming nonstop. Not only were they seeking advice from a neutral and knowledgeable source, but one thing became clear: As much as they wanted to believe their own dentist, they weren't sure they could trust the message—and a single resource to find answers to their questions didn't exist.

One person asked how she could be sure the crown that was recommended was really necessary. Another wanted to know what he could do about his puffy and bleeding gums. A third person asked when her child should have braces, because it seemed like every other kid in the third grade already had them. And on and on.

I returned to my book project with renewed determination and vigor.

Nothing But the Tooth is a reference guide that provides current and concise information on all things dental. Full of practical insights, it begins with how to choose a competent and ethical dentist and ends with a discussion about technological advances in the dental field. It touches on the high cost of dental treatment, pediatric and geriatric dental needs, the compelling link between your mouth and systemic diseases—and so much more.

This book will empower any dental patient—and that should include everyone—with greater understanding about dental health and procedures. In these pages, you'll find all the information you need to help you ask relevant questions about your treatment. After all, it's your mouth—and your good overall health.

❶

HOW DO I FIND—AND KEEP—A GOOD DENTIST?

Finding a new dentist can be scary. The relationship with your dentist is an especially close one, because she is working inches from your body. You're vulnerable, and with your mouth propped open, sometimes powerless to even speak up. Choosing one can be a leap of faith. Recently, both my ophthalmologist and my family practice physician asked for a dental referral. Makes sense, right? Ask a dentist if she knows a good dentist.

When I first began practicing, many patients sought me out because I am a woman. When I searched for a practice to buy in the 1980s, virtually all the sellers were male, predominantly white, and much older. Not only was the equipment outdated, but the decor felt stale. Mostly I didn't think the patients would accept me, a young woman, as a substitute for their longtime dentist. So instead I started my own practice. Since then, dentist demographics have changed substantially. By 2018–2019, more than half the dental students in the United States were female. In 2018, 32 percent of dentists identified as women and 28 percent as minorities.[1]

In an average year, you might be one of the almost half the population who visits a dentist[2]—and today you have a lot more options. Let's consider what attributes you might expect from your new dentist. At a minimum, you'd like to find someone competent and ethical, with a friendly yet professional chairside manner. You probably also want a clean office, happy staff, and convenient office hours, location, and parking. You certainly want reasonable fees and maybe even financing options. Ideally, everything should flow smoothly, from making appointments to billing. Finally, you probably want your new dentist to be punctual.

What if you have special requirements? You may be one of the estimated 12 percent of the population that has extreme dental anxiety.[3] If so, you'd be happier with a dentist who allows more time to get acquainted, or provides TV or music, or hands you a stress ball. Maybe you're looking specifically for someone who offers nitrous oxide, an antianxiety inhalant commonly referred to as laughing gas. Perhaps you have disabilities and need an office that's completely wheelchair accessible. Or maybe you wear a denture or only want gold fillings; most newer dentists have little training in these techniques.

You may have insurance limitations and must pick from a list of dentists preapproved by your insurer. If you have Medicaid, it can be challenging to find a dentist who accepts it, and you may end up going to a large dental clinic. If cost is an issue, a dental school where you're treated by students in a supervised setting may be a good alternative.

HOW DO YOU START LOOKING?

Word of Mouth

Begin by asking the pickiest friend or coworker you know. Ask your physician. Over the years, I've met lots of patients through my various healthcare providers. Conversely, patients often asked me if I knew a good physician, or dermatologist, or even plastic surgeon. Ask a dental hygienist or dental assistant who's worked for multiple dentists. They may have firsthand knowledge.

Online Research

Search data and reviews are available on just about anything. With an online search, it's important to distinguish between advertising versus organic results. The dentist in the ad may be the best one for you, but he is paying for the visibility.

With reviews, understand they are anecdotal, representing individual opinions. It's also difficult to figure out if those reviews are authentic. Some sites, such as Zocdoc, charge dentists an annual fee to list their name and practice. Others, like Yelp, give the listing more prominence if the doctor advertises with them. So if you're choosing from a Zocdoc list, be aware that those dentists have paid for their names to appear.

As a general rule, people who pick their dentist based on online sources tend to be younger. As such, they may not have complex dental needs and might just be looking for someone to clean their teeth. If you have significant dental issues, I would advise against selecting a random dentist online based solely on favorable reviews.

Contact Organized Dentistry

Many dentists belong to the American Dental Association (ADA) and their respective state dental organizations. These are further broken out into local components—for example, I belong to the Western Los Angeles Dental Society. Contact your local dental society and get the names of a couple of specialists who work with many general dentists. Specifically, you can ask for an endodontist (someone who does root canals) or a periodontist (someone who treats gum disease). Call them and ask for some referrals. They will have direct insight into their colleagues' workmanship and ethics. A layperson cannot objectively evaluate a dentist's skill or competency, but an endodontist or periodontist, who has gone through the same training as a general dentist, can evaluate and easily identify an excellent clinician.

Ask Your Current Dentist

If you're relocating, your current dentist may be able to provide recommendations for providers in your new city or neighborhood. But understand that he may know the doctors he recommends only by reputation, or he may have gone to school with them. While he may be able to suggest someone ethical, he might not have firsthand knowledge of the quality of their dental work or how efficiently their practice operates.

If you live near a dental school and are considering becoming a patient of an expert faculty member, recognize that the faculty dentist wears multiple hats: researcher, teacher, administrator, and clinician. If you were going to get a knee replacement, you would probably want to go to the surgeon who performs them day in and day out. Ask the faculty dentist how often she treats patients. While there are certainly outstanding faculty dentists, they generally practice part-time and their schedules may be limited.

Come up with a list of several names. If you have insurance, you may want to check that any dentists you are considering are in your provider network. Their absence, however, shouldn't be a deterrent against choosing a particular dentist. (Insurance will be discussed in chapter 3.) Make a preliminary call to find out about appointment availability. Often an urgent dental need cannot wait, and offices may reserve time for emergencies where you will be seen in a relatively short time. However, you may find there is a three-month wait for a cleaning appointment.

WHAT TO DO WITH YOUR SHORT LIST

Read Online Reviews

Once you've made a list of potential dentists, now is the time to read online reviews. (Don't forget to check out the hidden ones on Yelp.) Look for any comments—positive and negative—that are repeated in multiple entries. For example, several patients may love the friendly and helpful office manager, maybe even more than the dentist. With the negative reviews, try to tease out the objective comments from the emotional ones. If multiple reviewers have the same complaint, though, it's worth considering more seriously. Taken as a whole, the reviews might give you some impression of the doctor and the office.

The Dentist's Website

These days, most dentists have a website, often with pictures of the office and information about the dentist and staff. Does the office contain modern equipment? Does it appear well maintained and clean? Have the staff been working with the dentist a long time? If the entire staff appears new, this may indicate high turnover—and a difficult employer. Of course, you'll be able to evaluate the office culture much better in person. But based on their online presence, do they seem cohesive as a team and happy to work there?

What if the dentist has no website? This may indicate that he is in the later stages of his career and doesn't want to invest the time, energy, or resources into creating an online presence. He may also be busy enough with his existing patient base that he doesn't see the need for a website to attract new ones.

Check the Dentist's Credentials

Each state has a dental board that should provide a means for license verification. Begin by searching the state's dental board online. Many are part of a larger governmental entity, such as the Board of Consumer Affairs. Through the dental board, you can determine whether the dentist has a valid license to practice and if she is in good standing. Have there been complaints filed or actions taken against her license? All of this is public information. (As an aside, just because a dentist is on probation, it doesn't necessarily mean you should avoid that practitioner, as there may be extenuating circumstances.)

Learn about the dentist's educational background if possible. Typically, this information can be found on the dentist's website. Where did she obtain her undergraduate and dental degrees? Approximately 12 percent of each graduating class is inducted into a dental honor society, Omicron Kappa Upsilon (OKU).[4] Perhaps she graduated at the top of her class and is a member of OKU, or she won awards for academic or clinical excellence. If so, this would enhance the dentist's credibility. However, an absence of such accolades doesn't speak negatively of the dentist. Some dentists receive their professional training overseas. They are often immigrants to the United States, although occasionally an American will pursue dental education overseas due to poor dental school entrance test scores or an inadequate undergraduate transcript. In order to maintain uniform standards, before being allowed to practice in the United States, the internationally trained dentist must undergo additional education and licensing exams.

Dentists are also required to keep current through continuing education, and there are many highly acceptable ways to fulfill this obligation. The Academy of General Dentistry (AGD) is one reputable source for lifelong professional learning. If a dentist has the letters *FAGD* behind his name, he has attained the status of fellow within the AGD and has completed more than five hundred hours of continuing education.

Does the dentist have professional affiliations? While membership in the ADA is not mandatory, about 80 percent of dentists across the country choose to be part of organized dentistry.[5] Many enjoy the camaraderie of belonging to and supporting the profession, but there are practical benefits as well, including opportunities for continuing education and access to good-quality insurance.

Some dentists are members of dental honor societies such as the International College of Dentists, the American College of Dentists, or the Pierre Fauchard Academy. These organizations focus on ethics, leadership, and service to society and the profession of dentistry. Dentists cannot simply join these organizations; they must be nominated by current members and meet certain requirements. By themselves, these affiliations don't guarantee a good dentist, but they may point to a high degree of dedication.

Conduct a Brief Interview

If you're still unsure, consider contacting potential dentists directly. When my children were born, it was customary for parents to interview multiple pediatricians and select one; that doctor would come to the hospital if needed after the delivery. This may not be standard procedure for choosing a dentist, but I once had a patient who requested an interview. I balked at the idea initially but eventually agreed to the meeting. Not only did this woman become my patient, but she and I have remained friends ever since.

Now that you've done your homework, it's time to make a decision. Trust your gut. If you like everything you've seen so far, make an appointment. Remember: You can always change your mind once you meet the dentist if you realize it's not a good match.

PREPARING FOR YOUR FIRST VISIT

Because an appointment is for a limited period of time, it's helpful to take steps in advance to make this time more productive and efficient. This includes gathering pertinent information and prioritizing your agenda with the dentist.

Do the Boring Stuff

If you can, fill out any patient intake forms beforehand. Many offices provide downloadable forms on their website. If you have dental insurance, the office may ask for the information before your visit. Regardless, bring your insurance card with you. Also bring along a photo ID, as many offices will photocopy it for their records.

Confirm the exact location of the practice and find out how long it will take for you to get there. While this may sound obvious, it's surprising how many patients are late for their first visit because they got lost or underestimated the traffic.

Get Your Old X-rays

Arrange to have X-rays sent from your previous dentist. If the X-rays are film based, allow sufficient time for the office to copy them. Some offices have to physically take the X-rays elsewhere to be copied. Rarely will a dentist send the originals. Don't call on a Friday afternoon to request X-rays for your Monday morning appointment.

For the most part, unless the dentist has a specific question, he will not need to review the records of all your previous treatment and procedures. However, if you have a complicated or extensive dental history, you may want to have the records handy.

Disclose Your Medical History

Disclose all your medical information on the forms. You may be wondering why—what does that have to do with being at the dentist's? While it's true that you may not need to mention the broken arm you had in middle school or the liposuction from ten years ago, some medical information is important for the dentist to know prior to treatment. This includes:

- Any recent joint replacement, such as hip, knee, or shoulder. With most dental procedures including cleaning, bacteria that enter the bloodstream may be harmful to your artificial joint. You may need to take antibiotics before treatment. However, the thinking has evolved regarding this practice, since the data have not shown that dental procedures are associated with increased risk of joint infections. In fact, the ADA now recommends against routine antibiotic prophylaxis. Regardless, this remains a judgement call between the orthopedic surgeon and dentist.
- A prosthetic heart valve, heart transplant, previous history of heart infection (endocarditis), or congenital heart defects. Antibiotic prophylaxis is strongly recommended in these cases.
- Allergies to any drugs, latex, or other materials. Informing the dentist of such allergies can prevent complications. Nitrile has replaced latex as the principal component of gloves, but latex is still found in the dental dams commonly used for root canals and other procedures. Acrylic is present in dental appliances, from mouth guards to dentures. While it's extremely rare to have an acrylic allergy, it does happen. Patients sometimes report an allergy to the epinephrine or adrenaline used in local anesthetics. Responsible for our "fight-or-flight" response, epinephrine causes the heart to beat faster and may increase anxiety. As epinephrine naturally occurs in the body, this is not a true allergy.
- Any immunocompromised condition. This encompasses anything from cancer to organ transplant to HIV-positive status, which may increase the risk of infection.
- Recovering alcoholism. You may metabolize local anesthetics faster, and the dentist will be alerted to administer more local anesthetic at the outset or during the procedure so that your visit will be more comfortable and pain free.
- A pacemaker. Certain dental equipment may interfere with the electrical current of the pacemaker.
- A history or current use of bone-building medication. There is a rare but increased risk of osteonecrosis, a spontaneous sloughing

of the jawbone, particularly with invasive surgical procedures such as extractions. Knowing this will help your dentist make better treatment decisions.

The point is that you don't know which information may be relevant. If there's any uncertainty, it's to your benefit to let your dentist know.

Remember that all medical information is confidential. At the beginning of the AIDS crisis, most patients told me immediately if they were HIV positive. A couple were hesitant but eventually disclosed their condition. One man said, "Oh, I was so afraid you wouldn't want to be my dentist anymore." I assured him that as a healthcare professional, I had a duty to treat all patients indiscriminately. What's more, we used universal infection control measures to protect ourselves, our staff, and our other patients. Then I put my hand on his arm to reassure him. Don't be afraid to tell your dentist intimate medical information. It will be treated with confidence and respect. He will not judge you.

List Your Medications

Bring a complete list of medications you are taking, including any herbal or over-the-counter supplements. Many medications have oral side effects. For example, drugs for high blood pressure will cause dry mouth, which increases the risk for cavities, indigestion, and acid reflux. Blood thinners increase the likelihood of uncontrolled bleeding. Medications to treat epilepsy can cause your gums to grow and proliferate. Other medications may preclude the use of certain anesthetics or antibiotics.

As for herbal remedies, we tend to think of them as "natural" and safe, but the industry is unregulated and dosages are unknown. A supplement like garlic or kava can interfere with blood clotting. If you are having gum surgery or a tooth taken out, the last thing you want is uncontrolled bleeding. Over-the-counter medications such as aspirin can also contribute to bleeding.

Plan the Conversation

During an initial appointment, the dentist may engage in small talk to establish rapport, create a comfortable environment, and get to know you as a person rather than just a set of teeth. But you don't have all day, and neither does she. Plan on controlling the conversation. If you have questions, pick the most important ones and don't be shy about asking. Let the dentist know if you have a specific concern regarding your mouth. A skilled dentist will inquire about this at the outset.

YOU NEED A MASTER PLAN

If you have perfect teeth and gums, a cavity-free mouth, and only need a cleaning once a year, you probably don't need a master plan. But for everyone else . . .

- Triage and prioritize needed treatment. Create a plan with your dentist that takes into account your health needs, your health goals, your insurance plan, and your finances.
- It's perfectly acceptable to stretch the work over many years. For patients with considerable dental needs, I routinely crafted five-year plans.
- Don't forget to include any necessary specialist treatment in the process. Discuss the merits of each proposed specialist and their status relative to your insurance plan.
- Take advantage of any available health savings accounts. Explore health financing if needed.
- Remain flexible as conditions in your mouth change.

WHEN YOU AND YOUR DENTIST DISAGREE

Let's say you desperately want to have your front tooth fixed. The mismatched yellow color has always bothered you, and your high school reunion is coming up, so naturally, you want to look your best. But after a thorough examination, the dentist tells you there's a large cavity in your molar that is at risk of getting infected and abscessing. He's doing his job: diagnosing the problems in your mouth. You hear the urgency in his voice, but meanwhile you're wondering, "What about my front tooth?" The two of you have a conflict—and a disagreement.

Sit down and attempt to talk to your dentist. Communication is key, and a breakdown in communication is usually at the heart of any conflict. Sometimes the dentist has no idea you're upset. When I was involved with peer review, a conflict resolution program through the California Dental Association (CDA), it was not unusual for a dentist to be surprised by a complaint, believing the patient was completely satisfied. The dentist might simply be unperceptive and not pick up on your negative vibe. Perhaps the office is extremely busy and fails to follow through on unresolved situations, or the office manager thinks she is shielding the dentist from bad news and neglects to inform him.

In this particular situation, he may not understand the significance of the front tooth's appearance to you. After communicating your concerns, one of several things may happen:

- He may object, saying it would be unethical of him to address a cosmetic concern when your health is at stake.
- You may agree to proceed with fixing the cavity provided he do something temporarily to improve the front tooth.
- He may compromise, agreeing to remove the cavity in the molar and place a temporary filling, then fix your front tooth.
- You may conclude that the two of you will not be a good fit and decide to start afresh with a new dentist.

SWITCHING DENTISTS

When you change dentists, you are entitled to a copy of your records. This includes everything from X-rays to clinical notes, billing history, and even photographs and models—plaster replicas made from impressions—of your mouth. The dentist must provide this in a timely manner even if you still have an outstanding balance. The office is within its rights to charge you a reasonable fee for this service.

Sometimes it's when you change dentists that you're alerted to a problem. Dr. New says you have five cavities, and you'll wonder why your previous dentist never mentioned anything. But who do you believe: Dr. New or the dentist you've had since childhood? Since you yourself are not a dentist, how can you tell if the information is accurate? The majority of dentists are honest professionals who want to do the right thing. There are also innumerable subtleties and judgement calls in diagnosis and treatment options. If you ask ten dentists, you may get ten different opinions. If you get divergent diagnoses, consider a neutral third opinion. Tell Dr. Number Three you are there only to get an evaluation; you have no intention of becoming her patient or getting any dental work done. You may get the most honest appraisal of your mouth this way.

In heavily populated urban centers, the environment is competitive, and many communities have an abundance of dentists. In a state like Washington, there may be sixty-five dentists for each hundred thousand people, yet in Alabama that number drops by more than half, to only thirty dentists.[6] If you live in an area saturated with dentists, be wary of the dentist who cleverly picks up on your dissatisfaction with your previous dentist. He may agree with all your complaints and appear overly critical, motivated by the prospect of more business. Dentistry can occasionally be extremely challenging, and it is unrealistic to expect a perfect result every single time. Keep in mind that the chastising dentist wasn't there during the original procedure.

WHEN DENTISTS PRACTICE BAD DENTISTRY

What if you think some malpractice or incompetence was involved? Not only do you feel maligned, but you seek vindication. Furthermore, you don't want anyone else to undergo the same traumatic experience. What are your options?

Post a Review

Consider posting a negative review. Like the world's ever-expanding pile of plastic, we all know that information on the internet stays out there for a very long time. So keep this in mind before you post: A less-than-ideal outcome does not mean your dentist did anything wrong. She may have followed proper surgical protocol, but your implant still fell out. Maybe it had to do with your immune system, or you inadvertently chewed on that area and put pressure on the implant. Sometimes it's nobody's fault. Bad outcomes happen.

Frequently fault is impossible to determine, and it becomes a "he said, she said" scenario. In 2010, a dentist sued Yelp and the parents of a pediatric patient for libel, alleging that a review posted on the site was inaccurate and damaging to her reputation. The review said that the dentist should be avoided "like a disease." Without investigating the merits of the case, the court sided with Yelp and the parents, citing the California SLAPP (strategic lawsuit against public participation) law, which upheld the defendants' right to speak out on public issues. In this case, the issue concerned amalgam, the material used in silver fillings. The safety of amalgam, with its mercury content, has been hotly debated in the public arena and is considered a "public issue." Not only did the dentist end up with an $80,000 legal bill, but her specific objections to the inaccuracy of the review were never addressed.[7]

No dentist—or physician, or manicurist, or restaurateur—wants to go through this nightmarish experience. When an emotionally charged negative review is posted, the only recourse is to dilute it with more positive entries. Words matter, though, and they can ruin reputations. If you do choose to post a negative review, stick to objective comments wherever possible. For instance, you might say the floors were dirty and post a picture of the floor littered with debris. This gives the establishment a chance to rectify the problem. However, if you truly feel that the dentist is guilty of malpractice, there may be better solutions.

File a Complaint with the Dental Board

Each state has a dental board made up of dental professionals and public members. The agency governs licensing, establishes standards of practice and conduct, and takes disciplinary action when appropriate. In most states, you can file a complaint directly on the dental board's website. In 2020, complaints were down because dental offices were closed for part of the year as a result of the COVID-19 pandemic. In the fourth quarter of 2019, there were almost one thousand complaints to the California Dental Board. The majority of the complaints had to do with gross or repeated acts of negligence, incompetence, fraud, sexual misconduct, improper advertising, substance abuse, and substandard infection control protocol. Due to COVID, the public now has a much better awareness of proper infection control procedures, and it would not be unexpected to see an increase of complaints in this area.

The dental board will not make a ruling on your complaint or force the dentist to give you a refund. Instead, egregious cases will be referred to the district attorney's office for further investigation and possible criminal prosecution. This includes situations of sexual misconduct or insurance and other financial fraud. If action is taken, the dental board has the authority to temporarily suspend, revoke, or place a dentist on probation. The names are then published on the dental board's website.

Seek Out Peer Review

Another avenue for handling complaints is peer review. These programs were established by state dental associations as a means of straightforward, unbiased, and efficient conflict resolution. Although the programs vary by state, peer volunteer dentists evaluate the nature of each complaint. If the work is judged to be deficient, they will order the dentist to refund your money. You may be thinking that this is an old boys' club, where dentists protect each other, but that is not the case. In my decade as a peer review volunteer, statistics indicated that every year, cases were evenly split in favor of the patient or the dentist.

Sadly, over the last several years, many state dental associations have dropped or defunded their peer review programs. These programs provide a valuable service for both patients and dentists. Hopefully they will make a comeback.

Consider Legal Remedies

Small claims court may be an alternative to peer review. This may be a quicker and less costly legal option than outright litigation. Claim maximums differ by state, usually ranging anywhere from $2,500 to $10,000. The judge will likely be a former attorney with no medical expertise. In small claims court, both parties usually represent themselves, and the judgement is in monetary terms; in other words, the judge cannot order the dentist to apologize for his mistakes.

Arbitration is another conflict resolution method; in this case, both parties agree to utilize the services of a neutral third-party arbitrator. Sometimes, as a condition to becoming a patient, you have to sign an agreement that prioritizes arbitration over litigation. In arbitration, the professional arbitrator has the final say on the outcome of the conflict.

Finally, you can file a lawsuit. Most attorneys take on malpractice cases on a contingency basis, meaning they don't get paid unless they win the case. You may be hard pressed to find a lawyer to represent you for a filling that fell out hours after it was placed, but if your dentist failed to diagnose a cancerous growth in your mouth that is now stage IV or told you your gums were fine year after year and now you're going to lose a dozen teeth, that's a different situation altogether.

Regardless of which route you choose to address your concerns, all these scenarios are very stressful for the dentist—and for you. Certainly there are incompetent dentists out there who shouldn't be practicing, ones who deserve to have their licenses revoked. But by and large, most dentists want to do a good job for their patients. As noted earlier, communication is often the key to avoiding problems.

DENTAL EMERGENCIES

Dental emergencies can occur at any time, and while there may not be a legal requirement, dentists are ethically obligated to make reasonable arrangements for emergency care for their patients of record. This means that when you call on a Sunday, the office voicemail message should include a way of reaching your dentist in the case of an emergency. (I wouldn't go to a dentist who didn't offer this service.)

Many dentists go out of their way to assist patients after hours. They consider this an aspect of patient care that is part of the job. Even though I could have charged an after-hours fee, I never did. You may discover many dentists are equally generous with their time. But what exactly constitutes a dental emergency? Years ago, I had a patient who called me at 10 p.m. because she was experiencing a "flossing emergency." Relieved that she couldn't see me rolling my eyes, I listened to her concerns. Her gum would not stop bleeding, and she didn't know what to do. I advised her to put pressure on the area, to avoid brushing or chewing there, and to call me the next day if the problem persisted. On the surface, it seemed like she was taking advantage by contacting me so late over a trivial matter. But was it? Clearly she was worried and uncertain how to proceed.

Most patients call after hours because they're scared and unsure about what to do. Most simply need reassurance and information. Below is a list of the most common reasons patients call their dentists after hours, with a few "true" emergencies thrown in.

"I have a toothache."

It's rumored that the pain of a toothache is worse than that of childbirth. Although I've never experienced such a toothache, I almost always make a special trip to the office to see these patients. Sometimes it's treatable. Other times the tooth is infected and the infection must be attended to with antibiotics before the tooth can even be touched.

Before the opioid crisis and the tightening of prescription regulations, patients would call on nights and weekends complaining of a toothache. In reality, they were seeking drugs. They invented detailed accounts of our previous interactions while I struggled to remember exactly who they were. I got wise to this tactic after the first couple ruses and would say, "I don't remember who you are. You'll have to come into the office for an exam first." Most times the only response to this was a dial tone. It's no wonder dentists are leery of unknown patients claiming to have a toothache.

There are legitimate toothache emergencies for which I've gone into the office on a night or weekend. If I discover that the toothache was a result of an ignored treatment recommendation, I try to resist the "I told you so" lecture. The priority is to take the patient out of pain.

"My mouth is swelling."

Swelling can be caused by anything from a wayward popcorn kernel to a life-threatening infection. If you're unsure, contact your dentist. She may ask if you're having difficulty breathing, if your eye is swollen shut, or if you're feverish. A picture or video will help your dentist assess the severity of the situation. If the swelling is significant enough to impair breathing, a visit to the emergency room may be the first course of action.

"My tooth broke/my filling fell out."

A broken tooth or filling is one of the most common reasons patients call after hours. This can often wait until the following workday or even a few days after. It may be to your advantage to wait because the procedure will turn out better with the help of the assistant, who won't be there on the weekend or after hours. In the meantime, your tooth will probably be sensitive to cold beverages or air. That's normal. If the broken tooth is sharp and cutting your tongue, go in the following day and have it smoothed out. This should only take a few minutes.

A picture speaks volumes. Even before COVID, many dentists were using electronic communication to incorporate teledentistry into their practice. I routinely asked for pictures of the broken tooth. More than once, the photo showed a tooth that couldn't be saved. Rather than asking the patient to come in for an unnecessary exam, I instead referred them to an oral surgeon for extraction and a possible implant. Communicating with your dentist in this way can save you time and money.

"My crown or temporary crown fell out."

A crown or temporary crown that has fallen out can also wait until the following day, or even a couple days later. Again, the tooth may be sensitive to cold water and air. In instances where you can't come in right away, you can purchase an over-the-counter denture adhesive like Fixodent at any pharmacy and use it to hold your crown in place. If you do this, always take the crown out before bedtime. It may become dislodged, and if you swallow it or aspirate it into your lungs, it can cause serious harm. Never use Krazy Glue or Gorilla Glue to recement your crown.

If you know you'll be traveling with a temporary crown, tell your dentist; she may use a stronger temporary cement to avoid unnecessary trouble while you're out of town. Alternatively, you can postpone your crown procedure until a more convenient time.

You might be wondering why you can't simply forgo recementing the temporary crown. Your permanent crown will be ready in a week anyway, and you're swamped at work. Besides, it's not bothering you. The reason is that teeth, like water, can move into empty spaces. Luckily, teeth don't move as quickly as water, and on occasion, they don't move at all. But when the area that had been occupied by the temporary crown is suddenly open space, there's a chance the underlying tooth will shift and your permanent crown won't fit— or your dentist will ruin the shine and integrity of the new crown with the amount of adjustment required to make it fit. Worse yet, he may spend most of the appointment trying to adjust it to fit, only to tell you that the entire procedure needs to be redone—at an additional charge.

"My tooth got knocked out."

If a tooth has been knocked out, run, don't walk, to the nearest dentist. I've received this phone call twice during my career. Once was from the mother of a kid whose permanent tooth was knocked out (avulsed) in a skateboarding accident. Unfortunately, accounting for early evening Los Angeles traffic, she was at least two hours away. The other was from a patient vacationing in Italy. Both times I was helpless to do anything.

Time is of the essence. If this should happen, you have an hour at most to figure things out. Gently rinse any debris off the tooth. Do not scrub it. Place the tooth in one of three solutions: Hanks' balanced salt solution, pasteurized milk, or your own saliva. The sooner the tooth can be reimplanted, the greater its chance of reattachment, but even then, the prognosis can be guarded.

Once a woman from an African country came in about a swelling in her gum. When I peered into her mouth, I noticed the offending tooth was turned backward 180 degrees. I pointed this out and she laughed. She said the tooth had gotten knocked out during the civil war in her country. There were no dentists around or any medical care to speak of. She dusted the incisor off and stuck it back into her mouth. "That was twenty years ago," she said.

"I was in an accident and now my teeth don't touch together the right way."

Your jaw may be broken. Contact your dentist right away, and he will send you to an oral surgeon. If you have multiple injuries, you may be tempted to go to the emergency room. Provided there's an oral surgeon on staff or on call, you will receive knowledgeable care.

WHAT DENTISTS HATE

Dentists may not admit it, but some patient behaviors contribute to the burnout many healthcare professionals face. Being aware of these common irritants might help improve your relationship with your own dentist.

Last-Minute Cancellations

Everybody understands that cars occasionally won't start or children get sick. But if you habitually cancel appointments at the last minute, your dentist will be annoyed. At a minimum, you should offer to pay for his time. It's difficult to schedule a last-minute patient to take your place. If your dentist is self-employed, he loses money when he sits idle—but his employees still expect to be paid. If he's an employee himself, chances are his compensation is calculated based upon his productivity. We're all human, and sometimes emergencies make last-minute cancellations unavoidable, but your dentist may try harder for you if he knows you value his time as much as your own.

Broken Appointments

There's no excuse for breaking an appointment. An unacknowledged broken appointment sends the message that you have no regard for your dentist's time. If it's a legitimate mistake and you simply forgot, offer to pay for the dentist's time. Some dentists charge a nominal fee for broken appointments and last-minute cancellations. However, the amount doesn't come close to covering their actual costs.

Chronic Lateness

I had a patient once whom I adored, but he was always an hour or more late. To solve the problem, we began telling him his appointment was an hour earlier than the actual time. He knew it—and we knew he knew it. Once he even thanked us for helping him stay on time. Over the years his tardiness improved, and he began arriving an hour early for his appointment. I didn't like seeing him wait in the reception room, but it didn't bother him one bit.

Being late forces your dentist to rush through your procedure, possibly compromising the result—or makes him the bad guy when he tells you to reschedule. It may also make your appointment run into the next one, which is unfair to the next patient and to your dentist. It's also unfair to you, because you deserve the best treatment your dentist can provide.

Treating Your Cell Phone as a Body Part

Many medical offices prohibit the use of cell phones. In a dental setting, patients often use their phones to listen to music or a podcast while their teeth are being worked on. But this proximity to your phone doesn't mean you should answer it in the middle of a procedure. Not every call or message is an emergency; most can wait until after your appointment is over.

Ignoring Treatment Recommendations

You may not wish to fix that chip on your front tooth that your partner finds endearing. It's your body and your healthcare decisions.

But if your dentist warns you that a serious problem will occur if you don't follow through on his advice, please pay attention. If you suspect he's trying to scare you into agreeing to treatment, there's no trust in your relationship and maybe he's not the right dentist for you. Or you may have a financial reason not to undergo treatment. Discuss this issue with the dentist or the staff. Many offices offer either third-party financing like Care Credit or their own payment arrangements.

Sometimes patients wonder why a treatment recommendation is not mentioned at every checkup. Perhaps the dentist has forgotten, or maybe the problem wasn't legitimate in the first place. More likely, after telling you multiple times, the dentist concludes you're not interested in pursuing treatment and is reluctant to be seen as pressuring you.

Leaving the Practice

It is always painful for a dentist when a long-standing patient leaves the practice. There may be an inciting incident that "breaks the camel's back" and motivates the patient to change dentists. Usually the patient has had misgivings occur before this point, but may have kept them to herself. An astute dentist will realize this and deal with it.

But sometimes, from the dentist's perspective, it feels like a betrayal. He has treated the patient successfully for many years, maybe even bent over backward at times. And then, after such a long relationship, the patient is gone. Once again, had the patient and dentist communicated more openly, he may have realized the brewing dissatisfaction and had an opportunity to correct the situation.

Excessive Fee Negotiations

In some cultures and countries, it's customary to negotiate prices in all sorts of settings. In a US dental office, it is rare, although some dentists do offer a small discount for paying in advance.

Strong Odors

When your dentist is so close to you that she can see your pores, she will be able to smell—through her mask—that you haven't washed your hair in eight days. She may have sensitivity to your perfume or cologne. And the two glasses of wine and salmon you had at lunch? Yes, even after mouthwash, your dentist will know.

FREQUENTLY ASKED QUESTIONS

Should I go to the emergency room for a dental emergency?

Patients often go to the emergency room for dental emergencies because they don't know where else to go. Although the care is expensive, it's usually covered by their medical insurance or Medicaid, so the patient pays nothing out of pocket. Emergency room physicians, though, are not trained dentists and are often unqualified to treat dental injuries or disease. They end up giving patients prescriptions for antibiotics and/or pain medications and a referral to a dental clinic. For strictly dental needs, visit a dental office before the emergency room.

What if my dentist keeps me waiting?

No patient likes to be kept waiting. What if your dentist is habitually late? It may be that the first patient of the day was late, resulting in a cascading series of late appointments. There may be a lack of communication between the dentist and her office manager regarding the appropriate amount of time to schedule for specific procedures, or your dentist's inexperience means she can't accurately predict the length of a procedure or anticipate problems that will cause delays. Maybe an emergency patient just showed up and had to be accommodated. As with last-minute cancellations, things happen. But if your dentist routinely makes you wait longer than fifteen or twenty minutes, discuss this with the office. Everyone's time is valuable.

What's the best way to complain to my dentist?

Depending on your relationship with the dentist, it may be easier to speak to the office manager, who can then relay the message. Or you can schedule a time to speak directly to your dentist, preferably in a private setting away from other patients. Alternatively, a well-crafted email may suffice.

With any complaint, try to keep it factual and unemotional, particularly in writing. Your dentist may appreciate an opportunity to address your dissatisfaction. On the other hand, if your concerns are repeatedly ignored, it may be time to look for a new dentist.

2

WHY IS DENTISTRY
SO EXPENSIVE?

It's a misconception that people avoid the dentist out of fear. According to the American Dental Association, by far the number one reason for not seeking dental treatment is cost. It turns out people are more scared of the bill than they are of the actual dentist. My father recently had an asymptomatic infected front tooth that was diagnosed from a routine X-ray. The tooth needed a root canal, and the estimated cost was around $2,000. Surveys show that only 44 percent of US households can afford even a $1,000 unplanned expense.[1]

Is the cost of dental care warranted—or are dentists charging unfairly high fees?

A colonoscopy runs around $3,000, the same as a rudimentary pair of hearing aids. Yet we rarely hear patients complaining about the high cost of their colonoscopy. By contrast, hearing aids are not covered by the typical health insurance or Medicare, the federal health insurance for seniors and people with certain disabilities. The average person has to pay for their hearing aids out of pocket, and cost becomes a significant barrier.

Dentistry suffers from the same dilemma. Fewer than half of Americans have dental insurance, and unsurprisingly, patients with insurance are more likely to visit the dentist. Yet even with insurance, the out-of-pocket costs can be significant, making up more than 40 percent of dental expenditures, compared to only 10 percent of medical expenses.[2] Imagine if you had to pay $1,200—or 40 percent—of your colonoscopy.

On top of that, out-of-pocket dental expenses have increased dramatically in the last thirty years. If you paid $100 out of pocket in 1990, by 2017, adjusted for inflation, you were paying $160.[3] That's a 60 percent increase! It's no wonder you think the cost of dental care is high. Everyone agrees that dentistry is expensive. Yet it's no more or less costly than other medical care or even veterinary services.

In 2018, Americans spent $134 billion at the dentist, representing about 4 percent of the total healthcare dollars spent in the United States. As the population ages, the rising cohort of geriatric baby boomers will require more dental treatment, so this figure is expected to increase to $203 billion by 2027.[4]

WHAT FACTORS CONTRIBUTE TO THE COST OF DENTISTRY?

Dentist Compensation

You may assume that a dental degree is a ticket to financial security. For the majority of dentists, this career provides a comfortable lifestyle that may include homeownership, overseas vacations, and country club memberships. But I have never met a dentist who picked dentistry solely as a means to get rich. Quite honestly, there are other, less physically taxing paths with a lower point of entry that don't require years of schooling. In fact, adjusted for inflation, the average net income for dentists has declined since 2005.[5] Even as dental costs increase, dentists themselves are taking home less money.

Dental Education

When dental education first began in the United States in the 1800s, the curriculum was all of four months. Today, almost all dental schools require four years' attendance, and practically every dental student has an undergraduate degree. Upon graduating from dental school, many general dentists continue their education with a one- or two-year residency.

When I attended a state dental school in the early 1980s, I paid the same registration fee as the undergraduates, less than $1,000 per year. The most expensive part of my education was the mandatory dental kit containing instruments we could use throughout our career as well as a supply of dental gold to learn how to make crowns. Today, most state universities receive considerably reduced government funding, and in response, many have privatized their professional schools in business, law, and healthcare. Tuition and related educational costs at UCLA Dental School are around $47,000 per year for a California resident and $58,000 annually for an out-of-state resident. At private institutions, annual dental school tuition and educational costs can range from $60,000 to as high as $120,000.[6] The price tag for a dental education is the highest in any of the healthcare disciplines.

After I graduated, I immediately went to work in private practice. Nowadays, not only is the financial burden greater, but dental students are getting less clinical training. In an effort to gain more training, new dentist graduates decide to complete a residency for further experience and improved confidence. If a dentist wishes to specialize, that's another two to five years of training. As a result, a newly minted dentist will have spent a minimum of eight years or as many as thirteen years in higher education.

Young dentists routinely graduate with hundreds of thousands of dollars in student loan debt. Like a mortgage, this obligation can take decades to pay off, and it impacts their every decision, including whether to open or purchase a practice, start a family, or buy a home.

Continuing Education

Practicing dentists are required to keep up with advances through continuing education courses. Requirements vary by state. With the exception of Wyoming, which only has a CPR license requirement, hours per year range from a low of ten in Indiana to a high of thirty in Kansas. There are free options for continuing education, often sponsored by dental product manufacturers. But worthwhile, unbiased education costs money, may involve travel, and takes the dentist out

of her productive practice. The best dentists exceed the state requirements and seek out high-quality sources for learning. Not only does
this benefit their patients, but it keeps them invigorated and excited
about their profession.

Changing Practice Models

In the past, the goal of most dentists was to have their own office,
where they could independently control their schedules, practice
philosophies, and life. It's one of the reasons I was drawn to dentistry.
Some dentists still aspire to be solo private practitioners, but the costs
and complexities of establishing and maintaining a solo practice have
become increasingly burdensome. In 2005, 44 percent of dentists
under the age of thirty-five owned their own practice. By 2019, that
number had declined to 25.1 percent. Older dentists, aged fifty-five
to sixty-four, still owned solo practices at rates above 60 percent. For
reasons that may involve family demands or work-life balance, female
dentists were less likely than their male counterparts to own a practice. Only one of every two dentists worked alone.[7]

As a compromise between owning a solo practice and working as an
employee, some dentists band together to form group practices. Many
of these are cost-sharing arrangements rather than true partnerships, aimed at reducing fixed overhead expenses. Some are specialty
groups, such as oral surgeons, where partnering together helps with
obligations like after-hours emergency coverage.

Dental service organizations (DSOs), or what some refer to as cor-
porate dentistry, are rising in popularity, particularly among younger
dentists. In this model, your dentist is an employee whose primary responsibility is to focus on patient treatment, while someone else takes
care of the management of the practice. It's estimated that about 10
percent of dentists work for a DSO. Among dentists under thirty-five,
that figure increases to 18 percent;[8] younger dentists with significant
student loan payments are understandably reluctant to take on more
debt to open their own practice. While some DSOs are dentist owned,
private equity firms have steadily entered this arena, attracted by the
profit potential. Depending on the state, DSOs can make up a sizeable portion of dental offices, from more than 18 percent in Arizona

to less than 2 percent in Hawaii.[9] By all accounts, this is a growing segment of dental care.

What do these different practice models mean to you—and to the cost of dental care? Being a DSO employee sounds attractive: The dentist just shows up and does the dentistry and lets someone else worry about everything else. However, as an employee, your dentist may not have the freedom to set fees, give discounts, or do pro bono work. Further, she may be asked to prioritize profitability. If there's a choice between two different procedures where one will generate more revenue, she may be advised which to select. Conversely, if your dentist is a solo practitioner or part of a group, he may have little flexibility in his fees simply because his fixed costs may be higher. He won't qualify for quantity discounts on supplies that a larger operation might enjoy. As such, he can't pass on those savings to patients in the form of lower fees.

Increasing Office Overhead

Whether large or small, various sources estimate that the typical dental practice has around a 60 to 65 percent overhead.[10] This means that for every $10 collected, the practice makes a profit of $3.50 to $4.00. The dentist's compensation, from which he must pay individual taxes, comes out of this. So does any reinvesting into the practice, such as upgrading to newer technology.

Traditionally, personnel costs make up a large portion of the overhead expenses. Besides salaries, there are employer tax contributions and employee benefits. There's mandated training on everything from sexual harassment to OSHA regulations to CPR. Rent accounts for another significant expense. If your dentist owns the building, there's the mortgage, building maintenance, insurance, and capital improvements (things like a new roof). Then there's the rest of it: utilities, office expenses, dental equipment and supplies—all the moving parts that go into running a business.

But there's more. Transitioning to digital X-rays means new equipment, computers, software, and training, not to mention cybersecurity measures for operations and storage of data. This technology makes dentistry more precise and user friendly, but it also comes with a significant startup investment, in terms of both time and money. Increasingly stringent infection control protocols translate to increased costs. For example, more drills (handpieces) have to be acquired so each can be sterilized after use. When I first started practicing, believe it or not, I worked in an office that reused its plastic suction products. They were placed in a cold sterile solution that obviously didn't eliminate all the bacteria, viruses, and spores. Today, everything is either single use or sterilized in an autoclave.

With COVID-19, personal protective equipment (PPE) shortages created a spike in PPE prices. The same box of gloves that sold for $6 before the pandemic is now $20. Many offices added plexiglass barriers, HEPA filters, UV light machines, and even extensive improvements to their HVAC systems. To recoup a portion of these costs, some dentists began charging their patients a nominal PPE fee, which was often met with resistance.

It's no wonder dentists are reporting more stress than ever, with many opting for the more carefree lifestyle of an employee.

Different Fee Structures

Regardless of the practice model, there may be several different prices for a certain procedure. If your dentist has agreed to accept a particular insurance plan, a filling may be $150 under that contract. The same filling may be $200 under Delta Dental, the nation's largest dental insurance provider. To complicate matters, father and son may practice together. The son's Delta Dental fee for the filling may be $200, but the father's fee under Delta Dental might be $270 because the father participates in an older Delta plan that's no longer available to younger dentists. And the fee for the same filling for a patient without any insurance may be a whopping $350. If you think that makes no sense and seems unfair, you're absolutely right.

This range of fees can best be explained using the airplane ticket model. If all the seats on the plane were nonrefundable economy, the airline would lose money on the flight. But if the airline adds a dozen first-class tickets and charges ten times the economy fare, then the flight will be profitable. In other words, the higher fare paid by the first-class passengers helps offset the loss of the economy fares. In the same way, when your dentist accepts a lower contractual fee with an insurance company, he makes up for it by charging a much higher fee to another patient. Sometimes, because insurance is so restrictive, the patient who ends up paying the highest fee is the one who doesn't have insurance and is paying 100 percent out of pocket.

More than ever, insurance plans with lower contractual pricing are dominating the marketplace. In an effort to attract patients, dentists feel forced to sign up for these plans. (Insurance will be discussed in greater detail in chapter 3.) Because of the lower fees, they try to make up for it with volume. Many dentists report working harder than ever yet taking home less money.

IS DENTISTRY—JUSTIFIABLY—EXPENSIVE?

Of the factors discussed in the last section, two stand out: The high cost of dental education, with its associated student loans, and the increasing costs of running a practice have contributed—justifiably—to the high cost of dentistry. But in exchange, your expectations should be equally high.

My daughter recently went for a cleaning and checkup. Afterward, she privately objected to the examination fee charged by the dentist, who popped in for a couple minutes and barely looked inside her mouth. When she asked him to check her mouth guard, he held it briefly in his hands and said, "Looks fine," without trying the appliance in her mouth. Granted, she was accustomed to her mother examining her in great detail—but no patient appreciates being charged for a service performed in name only. Should this happen to you, speak up and let your dentist know. You should always expect value for your money and a service competently and thoroughly performed.

Another expectation is transparency. Make sure you understand what you are paying for before the treatment begins. Some dentists will readily discuss this, but others feel uncomfortable talking about money and will direct you to the office manager. If the office remains silent on the subject of fees, bring it up yourself. It may not be a conspiracy to hide important information; they may simply not feel comfortable or be adequately trained to speak about money.

Sometimes a treatment plan changes midstream—or mid-drill. A cavity may be much larger than originally diagnosed and now the tooth needs a crown rather than a filling, at a much higher cost. Just like a home remodeling project, your dentist cannot foresee every possible course of events. However, the seasoned dentist and communicator should anticipate the most likely scenarios and brief you beforehand. At a minimum, work should cease so you and your dentist can talk about any change in the treatment plan. In my own experience, there were occasions when I saw a defective filling near the tooth I was working on. Often I went ahead and replaced the faulty filling without telling the patient first. When I mentioned it later and assured them there would be no additional charge, patients were grateful for the efficiency and the kind gesture. I, however, did not have enormous and looming student debt.

DENTISTRY IS UNAFFORDABLE FOR MANY

Although the expense of dentistry is justifiable, it remains unaffordable for many, including middle-income families. In dental seminars, speakers like to say that patients who truly value the importance of a healthy mouth will find a way to pay for it. But that pitch doesn't take into account the reality that there are millions of people who simply cannot afford to seek dental care. Roughly half of the adult population in the United States visits the dentist every year, but that number drops to 22 percent in lower-income populations. Children fare better, with six out of ten children seeing a dentist annually. For children of poverty, though, it's fewer than four in ten youngsters, and that's mostly attributable to the contribution of Medicaid, the government program that provides medical assistance to an estimated 72 million poor Americans. Across the country, 35 percent of children are covered only by Medicaid. In some states, that number approaches a staggering 50 percent.[11]

Medicaid benefits are by no means comprehensive, and they often fluctuate depending on the economy. During recessionary times—when low-income people may need coverage the most—Medicaid dental benefits are usually the first to be eliminated, particularly for adults. For instance, during troubled economic times, Medicaid may only cover front teeth. If a back tooth requires extensive restoration, pulling it is usually the only alternative. And despite the density of dentists in major metropolitan or suburban areas, many are reluctant to become Medicaid providers, citing the paperwork, endless bureaucracy, and low reimbursement rates. They would rather provide free services occasionally instead. In rural and low-income communities, there is usually a dearth of dentists serving this needy population.

Though not mutually exclusive, the other group that often suffers from dental neglect is seniors, primarily due to financial factors. It is estimated that close to 14 percent of older adults are edentulous— they have no teeth.[12] Medicare, the government-subsidized medical benefit for people over sixty-five, provides no dental coverage except in very limited situations. This is a shock to many seniors, who may have had employer-provided dental insurance. (Medicare also doesn't cover vision correction or hearing aids.)

Imagine you are an eight-year-old child with a toothache. It has happened before and is something you've learned to live with. As much as you try to focus in class, the pain nags, and you cannot concentrate on what the teacher is saying. When you get home, the pain in your mouth prevents you from eating a proper dinner. You try to do your homework but are so tired and worn out that you fall asleep. Your grades suffer. The teacher calls you "listless" and accuses you of not paying attention. It's like she has given up on you.

For this child, an easily treated toothache can have serious, lifelong repercussions. Students who fall behind in school cannot readily catch up to their peers, a challenge made more difficult by the negative reinforcement from being labeled as someone who doesn't try. If the teacher has given up, what chance does the student have? Added to this are the physical dangers of untreated dental disease. Infections can lead to hospitalization and, in rare instances, death. It's thought that Queen Hatshepsut, one of the few female Egyptian pharaohs, died from an infected molar in 1458 BCE. As recently as 2007, a twelve-year-old boy named Deamonte Driver died from a severe brain infection, the result of an untreated infected tooth.

Now imagine you are a senior citizen who has some difficulty eating, sees poorly out of outdated prescription glasses, and cannot hear. Maybe you also have mobility issues. You become helpless and isolated. Because your employer-provided dental insurance is now gone, you skip your regular cleanings and exams. A minor problem may become serious, resulting in an even greater expense. Perhaps you decide to pull the tooth instead. As the cycle continues, you lose more teeth. Eating is now challenging and painful.

Short of death, untreated dental disease is linked to malnutrition, heart disease, loss of self-esteem, and a host of other ailments. It—and many other conditions, from diabetes to COVID-19—dispropor-tionately affects vulnerable groups.

WHAT CAN BE DONE?

The hard, unfortunate truth is that there are no easy solutions. Dentists alone are powerless to tackle a wholesale reform of dental costs. Well-meaning dentists simply cannot afford to practice in underserved communities without some guarantee of income. And with a 60–65 percent overhead, the dentist who bravely charges $75 a filling will soon be out of business. But as a society, we must rec-ognize the real human costs of depriving our low-income population of fundamental dental care.

There are some ways for patients and dentists to reduce dental expenses, however imperfect.

Become a Patient at a Dental School

Some of my fondest memories are of the patients I met and treated as a dental student. Many proudly regarded their experience as a con-tribution to the education of a future healthcare professional. For my part, as much as I tried to live up to that potential, I was a student—and made plenty of mistakes.

The average patient at a dental school has more time than money. Each appointment can last several hours, and in that time, less den-tistry will be accomplished compared to a private practice setting. There's also protocol to be followed. For example, don't expect any cosmetic work to be done until your entire mouth is healthy. In ex-change, the fees will be approximately half what you would pay in an established dentist's office. If you decide to become a patient at a dental school, remember: Patience is key.

Use Medical Credit Cards

Banking deregulation led to the establishment of medical credit cards such as Care Credit. Today, Care Credit signs are in offices everywhere, from your veterinarian to your dermatologist. You can qualify for on-the-spot approval and begin your treatment immediately. Be aware, though, of the interest rates and the penalties for missed payments. In some instances, the whole amount will be due if a single payment is missed or late.

Take Advantage of Mass Free Dental Events

Many states or professional health associations sponsor free dental events, which usually take place at a fairground or convention center. Vendors donate equipment and supplies; volunteer dentists, lab technicians, and office staff donate their time and expertise; and community volunteers help with logistics and hospitality. Patients often travel far and line up in predawn darkness to ensure they will be seen. Generally only the most urgent dental need is addressed. Multi-appointment procedures such as crowns are not offered, nor are cosmetic or orthodontic services. And the wait times can be long. Be prepared to spend the bulk of the day there.

I have participated at these worthwhile events. Most of the patients had jobs; some even had dental insurance. I heard this over and over: "Even with insurance, I couldn't afford to get this tooth fixed."

Participate in Dental Tourism

Medical and dental tourism involves travel to a foreign country for complex medical or dental procedures, primarily to save on costs. In 2020, global medical tourism was estimated to be $11.56 billion, an almost 50 percent decrease from prepandemic highs.[13] But medical and dental tourism are rebounding and expected to rise, particularly with the support of local governments and continued patient demand. Mexico and Costa Rica have become the most popular destinations for dental care;[14] however, patients of mine have also sought care in India, Thailand, and Brazil.

For the patient, dental tourism can be fraught with risk, beginning with choosing a provider. What if a serious complication occurs, one that might involve hospitalization or further medical care? Will your medical insurance cover those expenses? Medicare, for example, offers no coverage outside the United States. If the work is substandard or something goes wrong after you return home, there is little recourse. Frequently patients must have the treatment redone at a higher cost than they would have paid in the first place.

Years ago, I met a patient who had a mouthful of crowns done in Costa Rica. While the workmanship was superior, each and every crown fractured and had to be replaced. The dentist in Costa Rica had chosen the wrong material, one that couldn't withstand the chewing forces of back teeth (molars). The isolated dental work I evaluated from Thailand and India was also problematic. On the other hand, some of the most beautiful dentistry I've ever seen was done by a dentist in Brazil.

Think Twice Before Going to the Emergency Room

Patients who go to the emergency room for a dental problem typically don't have a family dentist. Most have Medicaid and are hardpressed to find a dentist at all. Faced with the tough choice of seeking and paying for dental care versus an emergency room visit that is free with Medicaid and Medicare, patients will generally choose the latter.

Emergency room visits for dental issues cost the country more than $2 billion in 2017. In 2018, 42.2 percent of emergency room dental bills were billed to Medicaid.[15] The patients themselves, however, seldom receive actual dental care. They leave with only prescriptions for infection or pain and possibly a referral to a low-cost dental clinic. And the taxpayer shoulders the cost of this expensive and often ineffective route of care.

Individual Dentist Philanthropy

It may sound corny, but aside from whatever security the profession provides, dentists are drawn to this field because they enjoy being of service to others. Many dentists quietly perform pro bono work in their offices. They might extend a payment plan to a needy patient or discreetly forgive a debt. Some dentists volunteer or even pay out of pocket for humanitarian missions abroad, including oral surgeons who correct cleft lips and palates. Many participate in the same programs year after year.

One successful program to deliver free dental care to children was started in 2002 by two dentists, Drs. Jeff Dalin and B. Ray Storm, in St. Louis. Christened Give Kids A Smile and adopted by the ADA, the nationwide program now treats more than three hundred thousand children annually with the help of sixty-five hundred volunteer dentists.[16]

Corporate Philanthropy

Companies in the dental industry routinely contribute through their charitable foundations, often donating equipment and supplies to mass dental events and to dental nonprofits. In 2021, Henry Schein donated 2.5 million items of PPE to frontline medical workers in India and Brazil. Companies underwrite continuing education for dentists. Procter & Gamble, which manufactures Crest and Oral-B products, provides free education on a wide variety of dental subjects.

IF ONLY . . . SOME ASPIRATIONAL IDEAS

In a perfect world, you would be able to afford a healthy mouth, your dentist would be compensated fairly and commensurate with his years of education and experience, and lower-income people would have equal access to basic dental care. Unfortunately, we don't live in a perfect world.

Again, I ask: What can be done?

Expand Medicare

In 2021, President Joe Biden proposed expanding Medicare to include dental, vision, and hearing coverage. Replacing missing teeth is expensive, particularly any treatment involving dental implants.

A single implant and the necessary crown can cost thousands of dollars. In the minds of politicians and others, this scenario conjures up a flood of runaway costs. It's no surprise that this proposal met with resistance and eventual failure.

Mental health coverage faced many of the same financial obstacles until stakeholders presented an affordable middle-ground plan. Ultimately, proponents have to show that it's more expensive to *not* have Medicare dental coverage than it is to have it. Even the most basic dental coverage through Medicare could benefit many.

Establish Medicaid Clinics

Another idea is the establishment of Medicaid dental clinics. State and federal governments are already spending a hefty amount on Medicaid—to limited effect—so why not set up dental clinics within or adjacent to urban hospitals to treat lower-income patients? Dentists could be hired at salaries similar to what they might earn at a DSO, or partnerships could be set up with dental schools to provide training for students or residents.

Utilize Dental Therapists

We can also incorporate less expensive manpower in the form of dental therapists. Similar to physician assistants, nurse practitioners, or nurse anesthetists in medical settings, dental therapists can perform procedures such as fluoride treatments, sealants, and simple fillings. This is not a new idea, but it has met with repeated resistance from organized dentistry. There is fear that the use of dental therapists may negatively impact the livelihood of dentists. There's also concern that standards will be lowered or that less-than-ideal treatment will be rendered. But for the millions of Americans unable to afford dentistry, this may provide a therapeutic middle ground.

Despite resistance, since 2009, thirteen states have enacted laws allowing dental therapists. The most recent was Oregon in June 2021. During a ten-year period working with dental therapists, the Alaska Native community had better preventive care and lower rates of tooth extractions throughout the state. In Minnesota, dental therapists have been licensed to practice in underserved areas for more than a decade; in addition to holding a bachelor's degree, they are required to be licensed as dental hygienists.[17]

The groups that would benefit from the use of dental therapists are currently largely ignored by most dentists. For example, when my mother lived in a memory care facility, I would have welcomed a regular visit from a dental therapist. Not only would this practitioner have been able to clean residents' teeth, but she could spot brewing oral emergencies, apply fluoride treatments, and show the staff how to properly brush the residents' teeth. In the Medicaid setting, the dental therapist can lower the overall costs of providing skilled care. Dentists already utilize dental assistants to take X-rays and aid in procedures as well as dental hygienists to clean teeth, take X-rays, and discuss gum disease with patients. The addition of a dental therapist makes sense.

Improve Public Health Education

Dental education for the public needs to be improved. In my practice, I was surprised that many parents sent their young children to school with Fruit Roll-Ups in their lunch, thinking it was a healthy snack. After I pointed out that this food contained more sugar than fruit, the parents understood.

Dental disease is largely preventable. Proper diet and hygiene can mitigate genetic tendencies toward cavities or gum disease. Regular preventive measures such as fluoride and early application of sealants can deter decay. Education of young parents can set the stage for a lifetime of healthy habits in their offspring. Similarly, education of children can establish a foundation of dental knowledge on which they can build these good habits.

Public health education requires a concerted and sustained effort on many fronts. Dentists can contribute to this every day in their patient interactions. And if all dentists assume the role of educator, perhaps as a profession, we can do our part to control the cost of quality dental care.

3

THE CRAZY, CONFUSING WORLD OF DENTAL INSURANCE— AND HOW IT DIFFERS FROM MEDICAL INSURANCE

Imagine if you didn't have medical insurance. Chances are you would be living in fear that one health catastrophe might mean financial ruin. The truth is that most people—especially retired seniors, the unemployed, and children living in poverty—don't have dental insurance. From 2014 to 2017, 50.2 percent of US adults with teeth, aged eighteen to sixty-four, had private dental insurance. Interestingly, out of this group, 22.1 percent chose not to see a dentist and take advantage of their insurance benefits.[1] In 2020, 42 percent of all US dental expenditures were funded by private dental insurance.[2] This is consistent with my practice, where approximately half the revenue came from dental insurance payments.

Dental insurance didn't exist before the 1950s, whereas medical insurance has been around since 1850. In 1954, the International Longshoremen's and Warehousemen's Union and the Pacific Maritime Association (ILWU-PMA) approached the three state dental associations on the West Coast with the idea of providing dental coverage for the children of their union members. Thus began the first three insurance companies to offer and administer dental benefits,

Nearly from its inception, dental insurance was designed to help supplement dental expense, never to shoulder the entire obligation.

Yet somehow the public has come to expect that dental insurance *should* pay for everything.

Who pays for dental care in other countries? In the United Kingdom, dental care is part of the National Health Service, where dental expenses are almost completely covered, with some out-of-pocket expenses for adults. Yet 24 percent of adults receive some or all of their dental care through private dentists outside the National Health Service.[3] Canada has a nationally funded, decentralized Medicare system that excludes dental services. In Sweden, free dental care is available until the age of twenty-three; after that, it becomes the individual's responsibility. In Japan, since 1961, almost all medical, dental, and pharmacy needs have been paid for by the government.

It's clear that the role of government as a financier of dental care varies around the world. In the United States, through Medicaid, the government pays for the basic dental needs of low-income groups and poor children. For everyone else, if you're fortunate enough to have dental insurance, it will help pay for a portion of your dental needs.

DENTAL INSURANCE BASICS

Dental Insurance Is Almost Always Tied to Employment

As with medical insurance, dental insurance is generally offered as part of your employment package. The quality of your dental insurance is a balancing act between the benefits your employer deems necessary and the premiums the company is willing to pay. Your medical plan may affect your dental insurance; if the employer's medical premiums increase, the company may skimp on the dental portion to save money.

When you change jobs, your new employer will hopefully offer its own insurance benefit. If you're in between jobs, you can take advantage of the Consolidated Omnibus Budget Reconciliation Act (COBRA) to maintain dental and medical coverage. Paying the often significant premiums allows you to keep the coverage you had with the previous employer for a specified period of time, usually eighteen months.

Medicare Does Not Cover Dental Care

When Medicare was instituted in 1965, the decision was made not to include dental, hearing aid, and vision services. Dental care is covered only under very limited conditions—for example, a broken jaw suffered in a car accident. This usually comes as a shock to new retirees when their health insurance plan that included dental coverage is replaced by Medicare. They now must pay for dental care on their own.

It's Difficult for an Individual to Find Good Dental Insurance

Patients without dental insurance who need considerable dental work often ask how they could purchase a dental policy. Self-employed people also want to find dental insurance. But without the volume of a large employer, where risks are shared, it's challenging for one person to buy high-quality dental coverage. Most plans either have many limitations or pay very little compared to an employer plan. With the expanding gig economy, the market for high-quality individual dental plans may increase, forcing dental insurers to take this segment more seriously. In the meantime, you may be able to obtain group rates for dental insurance through membership in a professional organization. Another option is through the Affordable Care Act (Obamacare), but be cognizant of policy limitations.

Dental Insurance Doesn't Cover Everything

The coverage of specific procedures is determined by negotiation between the employer and the insurance company. For example, because medical insurance premiums increase year after year and employers want to control their costs, they may agree to a reduction in dental benefits in exchange for holding those premiums steady. The employer may reason that while all their employees expect cleanings and checkups, not everyone will need a mouth guard. So the decision will be made to let the minority who need one pay for it out of pocket or with their Health Savings Account or Flexible Spending Account.

Just remember that what's covered is not always synonymous with what's needed. You may need a mouth guard, but it might not be covered under your policy. In uncertain situations, the best way to determine coverage is with a preauthorization or predetermination, in which documentation is sent by your dentist to the insurance carrier in advance asking if a specific procedure will be covered. While there's no guarantee that it will be covered when the procedure is actually performed, most of the time the preauthorization is a reliable indicator.

Cosmetic procedures are not covered by insurance. If a person has a severe deviated septum such that he cannot breathe adequately, then a nose job may be covered, but if it is solely to correct a cosmetic defect, then the patient must pay. The same logic applies to dentistry. Since there's no health reason why bleaching is necessary, bleaching trays won't be covered.

TYPES OF DENTAL PLANS

With most employment-based plans, there will usually be a couple options: a more expensive premium one and a basic one. Remember that your choice is not irreversible; during a designated time once a year, you'll be able to switch policies.

Fee-for-Service or Indemnity

With a fee-for-service (FFS) plan, you have the freedom to select any dentist you wish. You are charged for each service the dentist provides, and the dentist decides the prices for each service. Unless the fees are exceptionally high, they will usually be accepted by the insurance company.

Here's an example: You have a cleaning done and it costs $125, a reasonable fee for your community. Your dental plan covers cleanings at 100 percent, so there will be no out-of-pocket costs. You leave the office paying nothing. However, if your dentist charges $200 for a cleaning, the insurance company may determine that's outside the normal range of Usual, Customary, and Reasonable (UCR) for the zip code and cover only $125, leaving you with a balance of $75.

FFS plans have the highest premiums. While the employer may pay these premiums, a more common arrangement involves employee contributions as well.

Preferred Provider Organization

With a preferred provider organization (PPO) plan, you will be strongly encouraged to choose a dentist from a list of PPO providers. In exchange, you'll be charged lower fees, typically around 30 percent less than if you were a cash patient without insurance.

You also have the ability to choose a dentist outside of the list. Since the out-of-network dentist's fees will be higher, your out-of-pocket costs may also be a bit higher. Depending on the specific PPO plan, out-of-network fees are usually handled in one of two ways:

- *UCR:* The PPO plan will pay the out-of-network dentist according to UCR rules. Identical to the FFS example and assuming the UCR fee for a cleaning is $125, if the dentist charges $125 for this procedure, then the cleaning will be covered at 100 percent. However, a fee of $200 means the patient must pay the additional $75 out of pocket.
- *Fee schedule:* The PPO plan will pay the out-of-network dentist according to a predetermined and arbitrary fee schedule. Generally the fees are lower—sometimes substantially—than UCR fees, although once in a while, they will come close. For example, the fee for a cleaning may be $60 under the fee schedule and the out-of-network dentist charges $125. Even though the cleaning is covered at 100 percent, the patient will be paying $65 ($125 minus the $60 fee schedule rate) out of his own pocket.

With a PPO plan, the employee may still have to contribute toward the insurance premium, but at a lower amount than the FFS plan.

PPO-participating dentists tend to be ones actively looking to increase their patient pool; once they become busier, they may drop their least profitable PPO programs. When I started my second practice, with no patients, I signed up for a half dozen PPO programs. Within a few years, I had quit most of them. That said, today's young dentist probably has to participate in PPO plans to remain busy and productive.

Both the PPO and FFS models reward the dentist for procedures performed; the more dental work done, the more the dentist gets paid.

Health Maintenance Organization or Capitation

In a health maintenance organization (HMO), you will either be assigned a dentist or dental office or have the ability to select one from an approved list. Should you choose to go elsewhere, even if it's another dentist on the list, you won't be covered and will be entirely responsible for the fees, as if you had no dental insurance.

The employee usually pays the least toward the premium when opting for an HMO.

With an HMO, the dentist receives a small monthly payment regardless of whether you set foot in the office. In fact, there's a disincentive for the dentist to see you because in exchange for his payment, he is contractually obligated to provide many common procedures free of charge.

In general, the bulk of your dental needs will be met free of charge. However, there may be restrictions on certain services and/or copayments and upcharges. Think of the HMO model like an all-you-can-eat restaurant. You pay a set price and can return for seconds and even thirds, but there won't be lobster or steak on the menu.

While many patients are pleased with HMOs for their medical needs, my experience regarding dental HMOs differs. I've met very few patients who are satisfied with their dental HMO. The covered procedures are restrictive and upgrades are common, meaning you must pay additional fees. For example, a metal crown may be fully covered, but if you desire a tooth-colored crown, there is an extra charge. The dentists tend to be employees who come and go. Most are there to gain experience and increase their speed. If you find one you like, chances are you cannot request that dentist exclusively. My first job out of dental school was in an HMO office, where I was instructed to do one filling per appointment, even if the patient needed two fillings side by side. The patient was told to schedule another appointment—the first opening being weeks or even months later—to do the adjacent filling. It was an effective method to ration care.

DENTAL INSURANCE TRENDS

In the 1980s, some dentists decided not to accept insurance at all. They charged patients what they felt was fair and worthy, filed the patient's insurance claim, sometimes with an administrative fee, and expected to be paid in full; the patient would be reimbursed later by their insurance company. Many dentists who adopted this policy abandoned it later, after patients left their practices.

Today, FFS plans are declining, primarily because employers prefer lower-cost options. In California, Delta Dental, one of the largest dental insurers, stopped allowing new—graduating or relocating—dentists to sign up for its FFS premier option, instead directing them to join the PPO plan. If an existing FFS premier dentist moves to a different location—even if it is just next door—Delta Dental voids the dentist's premier status and leaves her with only the PPO option. With the PPO, the dentist now receives approximately seventy cents compared to the dollar she once got.

Traditionally the major dental insurers have been standalone, meaning they were only in the business of offering and administering dental policies. Now a convergence is occurring where medical insurers are offering dental plans as part of the entire health package. It remains to be seen how this will affect consumers.

In the face of rising health premiums, some large employers are wondering if they can cut out the middleman: the insurance company. By self-insuring, they save on administrative costs, gain more control over policy details, and may be in a position to react faster to an ever-changing health market.

THE FINE PRINT

If you've read this far, it should be apparent that dental insurance, like all forms of insurance, is complicated and full of details. In order to fully understand it, specific terminology and concepts must be introduced.

Preventive, Basic, and Major

Dental procedures fall into one of three categories, and payment is almost always category based. Preventive procedures, which include simple cleanings, most examinations, and most X-rays, are typically paid at 100 percent. Basic procedures include fillings, deep cleanings (scaling and root planing), extractions, and sometimes root canals, and are usually covered at 80 percent. Major procedures such as crowns, bridges, dentures and partial dentures, and sometimes root canals and implant crowns are covered at 50 percent. These are only guidelines and there are exceptions.

The Deductible

With the possible exception of preventive procedures, the deductible must be paid before the benefits begin, just like your auto insurance. Deductibles generally don't apply to preventive procedures, so if your cleaning and exam are covered at 100 percent, there will be zero out-of-pocket costs even if you haven't met your deductible.

Deductibles generally run around $50 to $75, although they can be higher. Sometimes family plans include a combined family deductible.

The Maximum

Almost all non-HMO plans have an annual maximum, usually around $1,500. The annual maximum is usually calculated on a calendar year timetable, but occasionally it's based on a fiscal year date.

When you consider that two cleanings, one annual exam, and necessary X-rays might run around $350 to $450, that leaves a little over $1,000 for actual dental work. If a tooth abscesses and you need a root canal—approximately $1,500 paid at 80 percent less the deductible—the balance of your year's dental benefit has been exhausted.

The crown required to protect the tooth after the root canal will be your financial responsibility.

Sometimes employers switch plans midyear. When that occurs, with few exceptions, the employees will start midyear with a new maximum.

The Copayment

The copayment is the portion of the cost of a procedure that is not covered by insurance and thus the patient's responsibility

Pricing Structures

While there are many variations on pricing structure, it is usually broken down according to the type of insurance.

- *FFS model:* The dentist may charge whatever she wishes but payment is determined by what is UCR for the particular zip code of the dental office.
- *PPO model:* Patients who choose a PPO dentist on the list will be charged according to a set fee schedule, usually around 70 percent of UCR. Patients who choose an out-of-network dentist will be charged whatever that dentist wishes. Payment, however, will be determined according to the specific plan, and the out-of-network dentist will be paid UCR fees or according to a predetermined fee schedule. Some PPO plans may also reduce the percentage paid or the annual maximum for an out-of-network dentist.
- *HMO model:* Patients are not charged for most covered services, and some procedures may have a copayment that is often based on a set fee schedule.

Dental offices are frequently told that fee schedules can be shared only with the patient, not the dentist. Unless you take the time to call personally, both you and your dentist are making decisions without adequate knowledge. Prior to any needed dental work, it's advisable for you to contact the insurance carrier and request a sample of fees.

Just being familiar with a handful of fees will give the dentist a good idea of how realistic the fee schedule is. Better yet, obtain a complete fee schedule if you can.

THE REALLY FINE PRINT

Waiting Periods

Occasionally there is a six-month or one-year waiting period before major benefits kick in. If the work is done before that date, the patient is responsible for the total amount. If the employer switches policies, the terms of the waiting period for the new policy will apply.

Pre-existing Conditions

Some policies will include a "missing tooth clause," a pre-existing condition of sorts where if you were missing the tooth prior to becoming effective on the policy, any procedure to replace the tooth will not be covered.

Replacement Restrictions

There are also time restrictions for replacement of work. For example, if you had a crown done on a tooth four years ago and you happen to need a new crown on the same tooth, regardless of the reason, the procedure will not be covered until five years have passed. Some policies have extended this five-year rule to eight or even ten years.

In situations where the crown was deemed substandard, with documentation that may include a narrative, X-rays, and photos, the insurance company may authorize a new crown earlier. Then they will ask for repayment from the dentist who did the inferior crown.

Implants

Implants have become an accepted and highly desirable dental treatment. Although their popularity is undisputed, some policies still do not cover implants but may give you credit toward the implant by paying for a less expensive procedure. Again, it boils down to what's been negotiated between your employer and the insurance company.

HOW DENTAL INSURANCE DIFFERS FROM MEDICAL INSURANCE

Dental Fees Are Not Inflated

My recent bill for a physical was around $700, excluding the lab tests, and my insurance company recognized and paid $269. The rest simply vanished. It left me speculating over the reasons why this occurs. Many assume that dentists, like physicians or hospitals, routinely inflate their bills. This is absolutely not true.

In my practice, patients tried to negotiate fees more than once over the years, but there isn't much wiggle room. Dental fees are arrived at logically and their value represents the amount of time, expertise, materials, and outside resources such as labs that go into a procedure.

Dental Annual Maximums Are Unrealistic

Most medical plans don't contain an annual maximum where, once reached, the insurance company ceases to pay until the following year. Practically all dental plans have one. These maximums, typically around $1,000 to $2,000, are woefully inadequate and have not kept up with either the cost of living or the cost of dentistry.

You Would Never Dream of Going Out of Network with Your Physician

The biggest difference between dental and medical insurance is the high cost of going out of network. For medical care, going out of network results in a substantial cost difference, one that could potentially put you in the poorhouse. Not so with dentistry! If you choose the PPO option and find you don't like anyone on the list, you have the freedom to pick an out-of-network dentist. Because your dentist will be charging undiscounted PPO fees, it's critical to know if the fees are based on UCR or a fixed fee schedule—and if it's a fee schedule, how realistic are the actual fees?

In a not uncommon scenario, your dentist decides to drop her affiliation with a PPO. You might share a special bond with this dentist and hate to switch but feel obligated to that of at least try someone on the list. The experience doesn't compare to that of your previous dentist, and you decide to return to her as a patient. While it will cost you a bit more, for many patients, this is a worthwhile affordable and realistic option.

PLANNING

Which Plan Should You Choose?

Given the choice between a premium and a basic plan, there are many factors that will enter into your decision:

- What is the difference in the premium between the two options?
- How much dental work do you anticipate needing?
- Will the treatment require a professional with more experience? In general, older and more experienced dentists are less likely to participate in a multitude of PPOs.
- Although this may be challenging to analyze, what is the quality of the dentists on each plan? Is there a marked difference between the premium versus the basic option?
- Is the work you need covered in both options?
- What is your overall financial situation? Financial decisions are not made in a vacuum; you and your family's needs must be considered in their entirety.

There's no right or wrong choice, or even a single best option. Much of the decision will depend on your individual circumstances.

Good Insurance Practices

On an ongoing basis, adhere to the following:

- Use your insurance. If you're lucky enough to have dental insurance, take advantage of it. Go to the dentist!
- Don't use the entire benefit too early in the year. Provided you have an annual maximum, reserve some funds in case you have an unanticipated dental emergency.
- Maximize your benefit. If you have pending dental work and unused insurance money that will be forfeited at year's end, schedule an appointment to get the work done. But don't wait too long. Many times patients call in early December and are disappointed that the month's schedule is already full.

Retirement Planning

Several years before you retire, schedule a comprehensive examination. You may be surprised at how much deferred work you've accumulated over the years. Once you retire, your dental insurance will likely go by the wayside as Medicare takes over. Remember that Medicare doesn't include dental coverage. Use your insurance before it's gone to take care of outstanding dental needs—and begin early.

Most seniors underprepare for their later-in-life medical expenses. Be sure to allot a realistic amount. Teeth may break. You may lose teeth and need to replace them. One implant and implant crown can cost as much as a luxury vacation.

CONSIDER THE DENTIST'S PERSPECTIVE

As discussed in chapter 2, the average dental practice overhead is 60 to 65 percent.[4] That leaves a profit margin of 35 to 40 percent, out of which the dentist must account for their compensation and investment into the practice such as new carpeting or acquiring equipment for new technology.

PPO plans generally discount fees by around 30 percent, resulting in only a 5 to 10 percent profit rather than the typical 35 to 40 percent. Most overhead, notably salaries and rent, represent a fixed cost. If your dentist charges $110 for a cleaning under an FFS plan, that amount drops to $77 with a PPO. Assuming the dentist's overhead is 60 percent, he makes $44 on the cleaning (before paying himself) under an FFS plan ($110 x .4 = $44). The overhead is $66. ($110 x .6 = $66). Under the PPO option, the overhead remains at $66 and the dentist only makes $11 on the cleaning. ($77 – $66 = $11) While the overhead can be mitigated by increasing volume, there's a limit to how many additional cleanings one dentist can do within a specified time period.

No wonder dentists are distressed over the decline of FFS plans. It cuts directly into their bottom line. The more PPO plans a practice has, the higher the overhead, leaving the dentist feeling like he's working harder than ever for less money. In addition, he may feel that he must accept these PPO plans or risk losing some of his patients. To make up for this deficit, some dentists resort to upselling, asking every patient about cosmetic procedures or proposing a more expensive procedure or material that's not covered under the PPO plan.

What about practices that accept HMO plans? The HMO plan is predicated upon two concepts, the first being sheer volume. The dentist gets paid a small monthly amount, usually around $10 or less, for each patient enrolled under the HMO plan. By itself, though, that's not enough to cover expenses, especially when most dental procedures are free for the patient. Second, HMO plans bank on the fact that not all enrollees will actually use the dentist's services. Even with those two assumptions, a practice that operates strictly on HMO plans will likely be a financial failure. In that sense, it's almost understandable that vigorous upselling occurs in this environment.

Ask the average dentist and chances are she will say she feels like a pawn in this insurance game. Older, more experienced dentists miss the time when they could establish their own fees without the interference of third parties. Younger dentists sign up for these plans because it's their only alternative—and besides, they have student loans to repay.

All insurance is complicated for patients and dentists alike. It's worthwhile to understand your dental insurance options and the details as this may affect your health decisions and outcomes.

4

WILL MY TEETH FALL OUT IF I DON'T GET THEM CLEANED TWICE A YEAR?

The dental profession has done a spectacular job of conveying this message to the public: Get your teeth cleaned twice a year to avoid any serious dental problems. Patients usually see their dentist more frequently than they see their physician. They look forward to the free toothbrushes and perhaps catching up on gossip with their hygienist. Insurance plans are consistent with this recommendation and regularly cover two cleanings per year.

But are twice-yearly cleanings really necessary?

THE DENTAL CLEANING

A cleaning, or prophylaxis, is the removal of plaque and tartar from the teeth and slightly below the gums, followed by polishing of the teeth to remove extrinsic stains. Plaque is soft, sticky, whitish-yellowish residue from leftover food and contains abundant bacteria. It can easily be brushed off. Tartar, or calculus, is hard, calcified plaque; it contains some bacteria. By itself, tartar may not be particularly harmful, but it can impair hygiene since it can't be brushed away, which can increase the likelihood of cavities and gum disease.

Local anesthetic is typically not required or used during a cleaning, but occasionally a topical gel will be applied for patients who have sensitive gums. Performed with either hand instruments called scalers or an ultrasonic device, cleanings can be done by either dental hygienists or dentists. With additional training and certification, a dental assistant can polish the teeth.

Think of teeth cleaning like house cleaning. It's something you must do repetitively. At regular intervals you—or someone else—vacuums, dusts, mops, scrubs bathrooms, and changes sheets. It takes a prescribed block of time and becomes predictable. The same goes for your dental cleaning. Most offices schedule forty-five minutes to an hour for cleaning appointments, which may include other tasks such as X-rays and an examination. The assumption is that the time allotted is sufficient to do a thorough job.

But what if you move into a new house and the whole place needs cleaning, from top to bottom? Not only did the previous owners leave unwanted items strewn about, but the house hasn't been cleaned in quite some time. It might take you days or weeks to bring it up to standards you consider livable.

The situation is similar with a patient who hasn't been to the dentist in many years. Maybe that patient is you. A simple cleaning would be inadequate to address your needs, and the work could take several cleaning appointments. (Unfortunately, insurance will usually pay for only one cleaning appointment every six months, so you will have to pay out of pocket for the additional required cleanings. After all, it's not your dentist's fault you stayed away for so long.)

The concept of a simple cleaning is invalidated when gum disease or periodontitis is diagnosed. It's akin to scrubbing the bathroom tile in your new house and realizing the tile has to be regrouted. You will need a periodontal procedure called scaling and root planing, commonly referred to as a deep cleaning. Scaling and root planing bears little resemblance to a simple cleaning and may take two to four appointments. (Gum disease will be discussed in chapter 10.)

Beware, though, if you are in your twenties and your dentist says you have gingivitis—inflammation of the gums—and need a deep cleaning, at an approximate cost of around $1,000. Gingivitis is technically the first, reversible stage of gum disease. We all have some level of gingivitis. Further, statistics indicate that people in their twenties generally don't suffer from periodontal disease, although there are rare cases of aggressive and severe periodontitis in children, adolescents, and young adults. Don't be fooled into thinking you need an expensive deep cleaning. Ask for corroborating evidence of your gum disease—and seek a second opinion.

But maybe you do need multiple simple cleanings. It's not uncommon for people in their twenties to forgo dental care during the post–high school or college years until they find permanent employment with benefits that include dental insurance. People of all ages can have a tendency to create abundant amounts of tartar in their mouths. Regardless of your age, if you haven't visited a dentist in years, you may need multiple simple cleanings. Rather than tell you only one cleaning will be covered, your dentist may couch it as a deep cleaning instead and bill it as such to the insurance company. It seems like a win-win strategy: You pay nothing out of pocket and your dentist collects more money, but technically, this is insurance fraud. Many insurance companies have become wise to this and request proof of gum disease in the form of X-rays and chartings. If you're uncertain, ask your dentist to clarify using the house-cleaning analogy.

Frequency of Cleanings

Returning to the original question: Do you need to get your teeth cleaned twice a year? In 2013, a study was conducted asking exactly that. It concluded that low-risk individuals are fine with one cleaning per year; their oral health will likely not be negatively impacted.[1] In response to this study, the American Dental Association said, "The key takeaway for consumers is that personalized oral care is a necessity for good dental health."[2]

If you're one of those people who loves getting your teeth cleaned, by all means, continue to do so twice a year. There's no harm in a professional cleaning. The enamel on your teeth will not be scraped away. If your insurance policy covers semiannual cleanings, take advantage of the benefit.

There are some patients, however, who should strictly adhere to the twice-a-year practice. There are even patients who would benefit from more frequent cleanings—three or four times a year. What conditions qualify as higher risk—and do you fall into one of these groups?

- *Periodontal disease:* Patients with gum disease, whether active or treated, should schedule their cleanings every three to four months, depending on their dentist's recommendation. Conscientious home hygiene is also highly beneficial.
- *Pregnancy:* The hormones associated with pregnancy can cause gums to swell and bleed more. Good hygiene and plaque control can minimize this, so it's a good idea to have your teeth cleaned a couple times during pregnancy. Some dental insurance plans cover more frequent cleanings for pregnant women. A word about dental work during pregnancy: It is safe to undergo necessary dental treatment during pregnancy, including the use of certain local anesthetics and the taking of necessary X-rays. The second trimester may be the most ideal time in terms of patient comfort.
- *Diabetes:* The relationship between diabetes—in particular, uncontrolled diabetes—and gum disease is complex. Diabetics tend to experience more infections, including periodontal infections. They also tend to heal more slowly. Advanced gum disease can cause a rise in sugar levels, further exacerbating the diabetic condition. Diabetics greatly benefit from quarterly cleanings.
- *Kids with braces:* Braces make it tougher and more time consuming to brush and floss. With the metal brackets, it's challenging, if not impossible, to diagnose small cavities between the teeth. Combine all that with a thirteen-year-old and it's a recipe for disaster. You may discover your adolescent has a mouthful of new cavities once the braces are removed. During the orthodontic treatment, schedule a cleaning once every three months. Purchase a water flosser and an electric toothbrush for home use to assist your child in dislodging food particles. Both will be well worth the investment.
- *Physical or mental impairment:* When someone is incapable of performing oral hygiene adequately, another person must take over the responsibility. Added to all the other duties of care, this

can be overwhelming. More frequent visits to the dentist can assist those with mental or physical impairments in maintaining good oral health. For those with difficulties with manual dexterity, a thicker toothbrush handle is helpful. It can easily be fashioned by wrapping duct tape around the handle to increase its diameter. An electric toothbrush may also be useful. Fluoride rinses can be incorporated as well.

- *Heavy tartar:* When I asked whether he smoked, one of my patients answered, "Every dentist I've ever seen has asked me that question." This patient didn't smoke, but he had extremely heavy deposits of tartar, even though he'd just had his teeth cleaned three months ago. It's unknown exactly what causes excessive tartar, but it's thought to be connected with saliva output. Behind the lower front teeth, where tartar tends to accumulate, sit the sublingual saliva glands. Another common trouble spot is the cheek side of the upper molars, home to the parotid salivary ducts. Patients with a tendency to form large amounts of tartar should get their teeth cleaned twice a year, or even more frequently.

- *Heavy smoking:* Some heavy smokers tend to develop a lot of stains on their teeth. From a cosmetic standpoint, they may benefit from more frequent cleanings.

THE EXAMINATION

What else happens during the cleaning appointment? For starters, you may have X-rays taken. (X-rays will be discussed in chapter 5.) You may be given a fluoride treatment. And whether you realize it or not, you will get an examination.

At the beginning of the appointment, inform the hygienist or dentist of any symptoms you're experiencing. It will alert them to check those areas more closely. A good practitioner will ask you whether anything is bothering you before you even open your mouth. The examination should be officially done by your dentist, but the hygienist cleaning your teeth may be evaluating your mouth throughout the appointment and reporting her findings to the dentist. The dentist will take a much briefer look at the end of the appointment. If the dentist is doing the cleaning, then you will benefit from her professional appraisal throughout the visit. Consider yourself fortunate that you have her undivided attention.

During the height of the COVID-19 pandemic, with more stringent PPE requirements, it proved too logistically difficult and time consuming for the dentist to pop in at every appointment. Instead, through a combination of X-rays, photographs, and reporting, dentists reviewed the information afterward and communicated with patients electronically or via telephone.

Regardless of the method, your dentist should tell you about her findings and explain them in terms you can understand. This is one of the most important parts of the exam. Was enough time allowed for you to ask follow-up questions? If further treatment is indicated, did she fully outline all the options, or did she dictate treatment and simply tell you what you needed?

This appointment is also the perfect opportunity to ask questions of your dentist or hygienist. Remember that time will be a factor and bring specific, concise questions. If the subject requires more in-depth discussion—for instance, you're interested in orthodontic treatment or ways to improve the appearance of your teeth—you can schedule a follow-up consultation.

The Comprehensive Exam

Performed at the outset of the dentist-patient relationship, the comprehensive examination for a new patient requires thoroughness, extra time, and expertise. You are paying for your dentist's considerable amassed knowledge and for the time it takes to discuss any issues.

Some dentists do the introduction, X-rays, and exam at the initial appointment and schedule a second appointment for the cleaning. Others combine everything into one visit. Still others schedule a separate appointment to present the findings and recommendations. Executed properly, a thorough examination can be an appointment by itself. Think back to your previous exams. Have they included all the following segments?

Evaluation of the Teeth Evaluation of the teeth includes inspection of individual teeth, in conjunction with the X-rays, for cavities, chips, cracks, or abnormalities. Any existing fillings, crowns, or bridges should be examined for defects. The teeth should also be viewed as a unit. Wear on the chewing surfaces of teeth, or on particular teeth, may reveal a habit of grinding or clenching.

With the aid of intraoral photographs or video, your dentist can show you exactly what he sees inside your mouth. Dental photography has become an essential tool in communicating information between dentists and patients.

Even with the most observant eye, your dentist may not be able to spot every cavity. Some do not appear on X-rays, and others are challenging to detect in the mouth. Your dentist will also not be able to predict structural problems. If your tooth breaks a few days after your checkup, you may be asking, "Why didn't Dr. Smith see this? Is she a poor dentist?" The truth is that dentists cannot see internal cracks within the tooth, nor can they tell you exactly when those cracks will break through, resulting in a portion of the tooth falling out.

Another unpredictable event is the toothache that's not directly caused by an untreated cavity. You might have a tooth that has a very large filling that was placed years or even decades ago. The tooth has never given you a problem. Then, abruptly—a week after your checkup—you wake up with the most excruciating pain. Again, you may wonder why Dr. Smith couldn't see this coming. It's not her fault. Any tooth with significant dental work can flare up at any time, become infected, and cause pain.

Periodontal Evaluation The periodontal evaluation consists of several different steps. The first is the periodontal probing or pocket charting, during which the dentist places an instrument in the tiny gap between each tooth and the gum to measure depth. Done properly, each tooth will yield six different measurements at various locations. Numbers below 3 millimeters indicate good gum health, and 4 to 5 millimeters may be areas of developing concern. Anything over 6 millimeters should be addressed. If the gum bleeds during pocket charting, that's another indication of periodontal issues. If pus leaks out during probing, there's active infection. A thorough evaluation also involves checking if any teeth are loose. Mobility is graded by classifications and should include an assessment of why teeth are loose. For example, all the teeth may be loose because the patient is a heavy clencher, or one specific tooth may be loose due to a bite problem. Additionally, receding gums should be recorded, along with the nature and quality of the remaining gum tissue.

Soft Tissue Evaluation   A visual inspection of the gums, palate, tongue, and floor of the mouth may reveal abnormalities. Red or white pigment may signal concern, as well as changes in texture, size, or color of a lesion. A sore that never heals definitely requires follow-up. Some patients have habits they're not even aware of, like biting the inside of their cheeks, which can result in unhealed gum areas.

The back of the throat and tonsillar area should be assessed for inadequate airway space. Further questioning regarding sleep quality and snoring may be indicated to assess possible sleep apnea. (This will be discussed further in chapter 15.)

Outside the mouth, masseter (chewing) and neck muscles should be palpated for any tenderness or pain. The temporomandibular joints (TMJs) directly in front of the ear should be assessed for the same, as well as any unusual sounds made while opening or closing the mouth. Clicking or popping sounds in the absence of pain are not serious but should be noted. A creaking sound (crepitus) may indicate arthritic degeneration in the TMJ. Any unusual deviation of the jaw upon opening or closing, either to the right, the left, or both, should be charted. An inability to open wide needs follow-up

Lastly, your dentist should feel for any swollen lymph nodes or other abnormalities.

Checking the Bite   An unstable bite, or occlusion, that can readily be tolerated by one person may result in agony and a complete inability to chew in another. Some things your dentist may look for include:

- Teeth that only touch on one side or area of the mouth.
- An individual tooth that hits first upon closing.
- Teeth that show unusual wear relative to the rest of the dentition.
- Extreme crowding of teeth that adversely affects good oral hygiene.

- Artificial teeth (crowns) done on implants. Teeth continue to move over one's lifetime, but implants remain fixed in the bone. The bite of implant crowns should be checked periodically, as heavy contact can damage or cause implants to fail.

Review of X-rays   In addition to looking inside the mouth, X-rays are an important piece of the puzzle in the diagnosis of oral diseases. With medical X-rays, your physician will refer you to a radiologist for their taking and interpretation. While there exist specialized oral and maxillofacial radiologists, your dentist is the one who will be analyzing your dental X-rays on a routine basis.

Oral Hygiene Evaluation   You may see your dentist a couple times a year, but each and every day, you're brushing your teeth. The dentist has an opportunity during the exam to see how well you're doing. He may point out areas that need improvement or suggest useful hygiene products. Try not to look at this as judgement. A good dentist or hygienist will provide helpful, neutral advice. Over the years I've been asked by patients, "Can you tell that I haven't been flossing?" It's as if they're confessing before being found out. The answer is no, I cannot tell what occurs in the privacy of your bathroom. I can only come to the conclusion that your gums are healthy and your hygiene is excellent. And even with superior brushing and flossing, some people's gums just bleed.

Evaluation of Your Appliances   All appliances need to be evaluated periodically because the conditions in your mouth change over time. Not only does this include mouth guards and retainers, but also dentures and partial dentures. Patients who wear dentures often mistakenly assume they don't need to visit the dentist because they have no teeth. But the gums shrink over time, and dentures can become increasingly ill fitting and less functional. Constant irritation from a loose denture can cause abnormalities in the cells of the gum.

People who wear oral appliances to treat sleep apnea also require a periodic assessment of the appliance, conducted by either your dentist or a sleep specialist.

Just as your teeth develop stain and tartar, your appliance may also be affected. It can be cleaned at the same time your teeth are being cleaned.

The Comprehensive versus the Periodic Exam

It's important to note that what I've outlined is a comprehensive new patient exam to be performed at the beginning of a dentist-patient relationship. In healthcare, we have been trapped for far too long in a paradigm that rewards doing rather than imparting knowledge and care. It's one of the reasons the United States spends so much on healthcare. Treasure the dentist who carefully and thoughtfully examines your mouth, and avoid the ones who offer deals on an exam that will often be cursory, or who walk into the room and begin the conversation with, "Ever consider a smile makeover?"

The Periodic Exam

The periodic exam is what occurs during a cleaning and checkup appointment. At a minimum, the periodic exam should include evaluation for and diagnosis of any new disease, whether it be cavities, gum disease, or a suspicious growth requiring biopsy. An examination of the teeth, the gums, and soft tissue should be part of the periodic exam, as should an evaluation of any appliances and the patient's oral hygiene. A normal TMJ doesn't need to be reevaluated at each checkup appointment, nor does the level of gum recession on every tooth need to be recorded.

A good exam may be even more important than the cleaning. For the majority of patients, an annual exam is sufficient. Even if you decide you don't need a cleaning because you rarely produce any tartar, go get an exam. A friend recently confided that her twenty-something-year-old relative's oral cancer was diagnosed during a routine oral exam.

There are some patients who need to be examined more frequently than once a year:

- *Children:* Children are a good example of a group that needs the exam more than the cleaning. They rarely develop the kind of tartar that plagues most adults. But between the ages of five and thirteen, with the exception of wisdom teeth, the average child will have shed and replaced their primary teeth with permanent ones. This process requires monitoring and, when necessary, intervention.

- *Teenagers with braces:* Teenagers with braces can benefit from more frequent cleanings and examinations. Many times I've noticed a missing bracket or loose wire and alerted the parent. A burgeoning cavity can even be treated in coordination with the orthodontist, who can temporarily remove the band or bracket, allowing access to the tooth.

- *The cavity prone:* Despite a healthy diet and meticulous oral hygiene, some people have a genetic tendency to get cavities. More frequent monitoring can identify decay in its early stages and prevent more extensive and costly dental treatment.

- *People with extreme dry mouth:* Saliva plays an important role in the mouth. First, it acts as a lubricant to facilitate chewing. Saliva also contains enzymes that begin the digestive process. It neutralizes the acidic environment in the mouth that causes cavities. Finally, saliva cleans away leftover food debris. Inadequate saliva results in dry mouth (xerostomia). This can lead to extensive decay, particularly on root surfaces, which are not protected by enamel. It also creates digestive problems and bad breath. Dry mouth is a hallmark of conditions such as Sjögren's syndrome. Many medications, such as those used to treat high blood pressure, can cause dry mouth, as do habits like mouth breathing or smoking. Saliva glands are damaged in head and neck cancer patients who have undergone radiation, leading to xerostomia. More frequent oversight in patients with xerostomia can identify problems in their early stages.

- *The elderly:* As we age, our manual dexterity and eyesight may decline, making oral hygiene more challenging. Gums may also recede, exposing root surfaces (hence the phrase "long in the tooth"). Cavities in the root areas present a challenge to any dentist. More serious concerns, such as broken teeth, may be present without the patient even being aware of them.

- *Heavy drinkers and smokers:* Though not necessarily related, statistics indicate that heavy drinkers are often also heavy smokers. All tobacco use, including chewing tobacco, poses a strong risk for head and neck cancers. Heavy alcohol use poses an equally dangerous threat. But combined alcohol and tobacco use multiplies the risk, which can be thirty times higher than in nonsmokers and nondrinkers.[3] In some parts of the world, betel nut chewing is endemic and popular. In addition to causing heavily stained and orangish teeth, betel nut is a carcinogen. The earlier a cancerous lesion is diagnosed, the greater the chances of treatment and cure.

- *People at risk for bone necrosis:* Millions of postmenopausal women, and some men, suffer from a reduction in bone density putting them at risk for fractures. Medications to combat osteoporosis, primarily taken orally but also via injection and intravenously, have been developed. A rare side effect is osteonecrosis of the jawbone, where pieces of the bone die and slough away uncontrollably, usually following an extraction. More frequent monitoring will reduce the likelihood that extraction is the only option for a diseased tooth. Intravenous osteoporosis medications are also used to treat certain types of cancers. The risk of osteonecrosis appears higher with this mode of delivery. Head and neck cancer patients who have undergone radiation therapy are likewise at risk for this rare side effect, termed osteoradionecrosis. For this reason, questionable teeth in the field of radiation are typically extracted prior to treatment with radiation.

- *The physically or mentally impaired:* Patients with conditions causing physical or mental impairment, such as advanced Parkinson's disease or Alzheimer's, are often unable to perform routine oral hygiene. Depending on the impairment, some may not be able to communicate any pain or discomfort. Regular assessment, even if it's not in a traditional dental office setting, may uncover dental problems before they become serious.

- *Bulimics:* The acidity of repeated vomit can deteriorate the enamel on the interior (tongue side) of the front teeth, making them more susceptible to decay and sensitivity. Because of their location, these types of cavities are also challenging to repair.

- *Meth users:* Methamphetamine addicts can develop a condition known as "meth mouth," characterized by blackened and rotting teeth. The decay is caused by a mix of poor oral hygiene, the acidity of the drug, prolonged periods of dry mouth, and a sugary diet. Meth users also have a tendency to grind their teeth, exacerbating the damage.

- *Heavy marijuana users:* The active ingredient in marijuana, tetrahydrocannabinol (THC), creates cravings for sugary, high-carbohydrate foods. Aside from weight gain, frequent snacking without corresponding oral hygiene can lead to dental problems.

5

DIDN'T I *JUST* HAVE
X-RAYS TAKEN?

Every day this objection is heard in dental offices across the nation: Didn't I just have X-rays taken? Instead of contributing to our overall health, X-rays are sometimes viewed with suspicion, that what we don't see can harm us. Sometimes patients think they're just a way to pad the bill. But the truth is that X-rays are an indispensable tool in the diagnosis and treatment of dental disease. Without them, your dentist would be navigating in the dark. The objective, though, is to balance the risks and benefits of X-rays and employ their use judiciously.

X-rays were discovered accidentally in 1895 by German researcher Wilhelm Roentgen. He announced this breakthrough innovation to the world with an X-ray image of his wife's hand. Roentgen went on to win the Nobel Prize in physics. The following year, American dentist Charles Edmund Kells took the first dental X-ray of a living person's mouth. Kells went on to become an enthusiastic proponent of the use of X-rays, or radiography, and even designed a device to hold X-ray film. Some early advocates of radiography recognized the dangers of radiation and recommended safety precautions such as reducing the amount of exposure for X-ray technicians. Unfortunately for Kells, after a decade of frequent and prolonged exposure to X-rays, he eventually lost his fingers, arm, hand, and shoulder to X-ray-induced cancer.

Despite the risks, the implications and potential of this new technology attracted widespread interest, from the military to Eastman Kodak, which became a major supplier of X-ray film. Dentistry was the first medical specialty to use X-rays in practice. The first dental X-ray machine, the Victor CDX, was developed in 1923 in Chicago. By 1932, 46 percent of new dentists surveyed said an X-ray machine would be one of their first purchases.[1]

DIFFERENT TYPES OF X-RAYS

You may be completely right that you had X-rays taken recently. But there are different kinds of X-rays, and each serves a distinct purpose. Find out what type you had previously and, as always, ask questions.

Historically, most X-rays have been taken inside the mouth (intraorally). These are the bitewing, periapical, full-mouth series, and occlusal. While the intraoral approach may be the most familiar, there are also extraoral X-rays taken from outside the mouth.

Bitewing X-ray   The bitewing X-ray shows only the top portion of the tooth not covered by the gums (crown portion) and is reserved for back (posterior) teeth. It is designed to check for cavities between the back teeth, which cannot be seen with the naked eye. It can also reveal substandard dental work in these difficult-to-access spaces. Additionally, the supporting bone level can be visualized, providing an indication of periodontal health. In cases of shrinking bone levels, the X-rays are sometimes turned vertically for a periodontal evaluation; these are referred to as vertical bitewings.

Bitewings are taken during routine cleaning and checkup appointments, and are often called checkup X-rays. A total of four is commonplace, two on the right and two on the left back teeth. If you've had multiple teeth extracted for braces, one bitewing on each side might be enough to capture all your back teeth.

Depending on your risk for cavities and the presence of existing dental work, bitewings are recommended every twelve to thirty-six months.[2] Barring any metabolic or genetic conditions or extreme lapses in hygiene, cavities generally develop during two periods of life and in specific areas on the tooth. During childhood, adolescence, and early adulthood, they form on the chewing surface and in between the teeth. As people enter into old age, roots may become exposed and vulnerable to decay. But if, say, you're forty years old and have never had a cavity or a filling, it would be reasonable to extend the bitewing interval to several years.

Periapical X-ray The periapical (PA) X-ray shows the entire tooth, including the root and the surrounding bone. It is used to check the overall health of the tooth, the shape of the roots, and the anatomy of the root canal system. The PA can reveal an abscessed tooth. In rare cases, a fracture can be seen from a PA, but the crack must be large and significant.

PAs are taken on an as-needed basis. If you're experiencing symptoms, a PA may show the cause. A PA may be also taken in preparation for a specific procedure, such as an extraction, where it is necessary to display any unusual root anatomy that may complicate things. Before starting a crown, the PA will determine whether the tooth is healthy enough to undergo the process. PAs are also used to check on the periodic health of a tooth or implant; for example, a PA is routinely taken six months after completion of a root canal to evaluate the healing process.

Full Mouth X-ray The full mouth X-ray (FMX) series is designed for the new patient when a comprehensive exam is indicated. It generally consists of eighteen X-rays: fourteen periapicals and four bitewings. The FMX checks for cavities, the condition of existing dental work, supporting bone levels, advanced tooth infections, and possible tumors in the areas surrounding the teeth.

Depending on the amount of previous dental work, the tendency for cavities, and the periodontal condition, an FMX is generally recommended every five years, with a range of three to eight years. This, however, is simply a guideline and dependent on each individual's needs. According to the American Dental Association, "A full mouth intraoral radiographic examination is preferred when the patient has clinical evidence of generalized oral disease or a history of extensive dental treatment."[3] An FMX is also highly recommended prior to any orthodontic treatment, cancer therapy impacting the head and neck area, or heart surgery. Sometimes an FMX is taken in the middle of orthodontic treatment to determine progress and assess the roots and bone level. Unless they are starting braces, children rarely need—or should get—an FMX.

If you are switching dentists, it's a good idea to find out the date of your most recent FMX and have a copy of the X-rays sent to your new provider. Side-by-side comparisons of FMXs taken over time can provide valuable historical information about your mouth. You may even consider retaining a copy of these for your own files.

Occlusal X-ray   The occlusal X-ray is the least common type of intraoral X-ray. It shows the teeth from the chewing surfaces and is mainly used in children when attempts to take either a bitewing or periapical view fail. The information gleaned from these X-rays is not as well defined. It may be used to answer whether a permanent tooth is congenitally missing or simply hiding under the gum.

Panoramic X-ray   Unlike the much smaller intraoral X-rays, the panoramic X-ray (panorex) is taken outside the mouth with a much larger X-ray. The panorex produces an image of the entire mouth, including the upper jaw (maxilla), lower jaw (mandible), and the teeth. In lieu of an FMX, a panorex is sometimes taken in conjunction with the four bitewings.

As the name implies, the panoramic X-ray provides a sweeping, wide-angle view of the lower half of the face. It's useful for evaluating jaw fractures, tumors, the temporomandibular joints, the maxillary sinuses, and the location of nerves. While it shows a big picture of the teeth, only large cavities will be apparent; smaller ones may be too indistinct to diagnose. Securing a panorex is customary prior to wisdom teeth extractions, not only to visualize the teeth but also to determine the proximity of the inferior alveolar nerve in the lower jaw. A panorex is also used to check the eruption status of permanent teeth and may be substituted for an FMX prior to orthodontic treatment. It may be indicated in the edentulous (patients without teeth) to evaluate the health and condition of the maxilla and mandible. It's often used as an initial screening for potential implant placement in edentulous patients. The panorex is generally taken on an as-needed basis. When it's substituted for a routine FMX, the same frequency guidelines apply.

Lateral Cephalometric X-ray   Used principally in orthodontics, this is an X-ray of the face and skull in profile. It's an effective means of planning orthodontic treatment by assessing and predicting future growth. Because of its three-dimensional nature, cone beam computed tomography(CBCT) (discussed below) provides a fuller and more accurate picture. However, the expense and radiation exposure are greater, and some orthodontists prefer the conventional two-dimensional lateral cephalometric X-ray.

Lateral cephs are also used to evaluate airway space in cases of possible sleep apnea.

Cone Beam Computed Tomography   CBCT enables three-dimensional viewing of an object. Because the format is digital, it's a scan rather than an X-ray. Just as the discovery of two-dimensional X-rays was revolutionary, this technology has been a game changer in dentistry.

There are multiple CBCT applications:

- It can clearly show the proximity of a nerve to an implant or a wisdom tooth.
- Undiagnosed tooth fractures may magically appear, some which the patient may have complained about repeatedly and unsuccessfully. After saying, "Something's not right," for months, imagine the patient's validation upon uncovering a fracture.
- CBCT is employed to accurately predict the quantity and quality of bone prior to implant placement, resulting in less failures.
- CBCT is used to show the complex anatomy of canals in a root canal procedure.
- It can determine the exact location and size of tumors.
- In orthodontics, CBCT can assess and predict patient growth.
- With gum disease, it can show the extent and location of three-dimensional bone defects so more targeted grafting therapy can occur.
- CBCT accurately depicts the TMJ for specific pathology.
- It can be used to locate a buried extra tooth (supernumerary), a broken needle, or even bullet fragments.

One area where CBCT is not used is to diagnose cavities. When a bitewing is sufficient, the expense and additional radiation of a CBCT scan simply isn't justified. CBCT is recommended on an as-needed basis. Because of the higher radiation, it should be used judiciously in children.

GOING DIGITAL

In 1987, Francis Mouyen, a physicist, introduced the first dental digital radiography system. Instead of using film, an image—the X-ray—is captured digitally and stored on a computer or in the cloud. Today, digital radiography has overtaken the conventional film-based method. (In an ironic twist, the first digital camera was invented by a Kodak engineer in 1975. Unfortunately, the camera was ignored by management as the company continued to focus on its film business, including the sale of dental X-ray film. Kodak's strategic blunder to recognize the coming disruption of digital technology led to its eventual bankruptcy.)

The advent of digital freed dentists from the messy, smelly darkroom where film X-rays were processed. Gone were the gallons of developer and fixer, along with the stubborn stains they left on uniforms. The space might have been converted into a storeroom—or, better yet, a spot for the new digital panoramic machine.

The software used to view digital X-ray images allows for image manipulation, much like the software used to edit digital photographs. Color, density, contrast, and size can all be adjusted to produce a more accurate and diagnostic image. The copying and sending of X-ray images are vastly improved. In the past, it was a tedious trial-and-error process to duplicate X-rays. Alternatively, X-ray film could be purchased with two films per packet so that a duplicate set of X-rays would be readily available. Now, with a few clicks of a mouse, entire sets of X-rays can be electronically shared with patients or specialists. But no doubt the most significant advantage lies in lowered radiation exposure: It is estimated that digital X-rays result in 50 to 80 percent less radiation than conventional X-rays.[4]

Converting to a digital format is quite a process, though. The initial cost of the X-ray machine, software, and computer hardware can be formidable. Learning how to operate the software in partnership with the machine and how to store and maintain images securely can also be a substantial task. Despite this, most dentists agree that the benefits—in terms of increased efficiency, better images, and lower radiation exposure—outweigh the costs.

TYPES OF X-RAY MACHINES

Just as there are multiple kinds of X-rays, different machines produce different radiographs. Most X-rays are taken in your dentist's office or at a specialist's office, but occasionally, you'll be sent to an X-ray lab or imaging center containing various machines for an entire workup. This is a common practice among some orthodontists who don't possess their own X-ray units.

Some X-ray machines operate exclusively with film, but most can be adapted to capture a digital image using either a bulky solid-state sensor—which you may not appreciate in your mouth—or a phosphor plate one that is similar in size and shape to traditional X-ray film.

Conventional Intraoral X-ray Machine

Attached to the wall in your dentist's office, this machine may have started out taking intraoral film X-rays. It can usually be converted into capturing digital images by the addition of a sensor, software, and a computer.

Handheld X-ray Unit

Initially developed for humanitarian missions and military triage use, handheld devices appeared in the 1990s. With a name like Nomad and shaped like either a camera or a hair dryer, they are an inexpensive alternative to wall-mounted units. Handheld devices can take either intraoral film X-rays or digital scans. Benefits include portability and cost savings.

With the operator in the room and next to the patient, managing challenging situations such as taking an X-ray on a gagger becomes easier. But operator presence is also the biggest drawback: Unless techniques are precisely followed and the equipment is well main-

tained, the operator will receive more backscatter and leakage radiation. Handheld devices are nevertheless essential to the success of
large-scale dental events where hundreds of patients are treated at
a convention center, arena, or the like.

Panoramic Machine

Most panoramic machines can take either panorex or lateral cephalometric X-rays. Additionally, some are upgradable to a digital format,
and still others are available in a three-dimensional format.

Newer panoramic machines are also capable of taking extraoral
bitewings. This technology is transformative for the many patients—
gaggers, children, people with extremely small mouths—who cannot
tolerate an X-ray inside the mouth. Many dentists consider external
bitewings less diagnostic for cavities because they look more like
periapical X-rays.

CBCT Machine

CBCT machines sell for a staggering $50,000 to $100,000 and occasionally more.[5] Before a dentist acquires one of these expensive
machines, he must decide whether he needs a CBCT for doing root
canals or for placing a mouthful of implants, because the machines
are very function specific. He cannot do both with the same machine.

Since they first became available in the early 2000s, CBCT machines have been primarily purchased by specialists, imaging centers,
and academic institutions. But marketing pressure to possess the
latest technology has contributed to the popularity of these machines
among general dentists. The next time you visit your dentist, you may
notice a brand new state-of-the-art CBCT machine. It's large and
similar in appearance to a panorex.

While advances in healthcare often involve embracing new technology, two problems have surfaced. First, for many dentists, CBCT
technology didn't yet exist during their training; even newer dentists
may not have encountered this subject as part of their dental school
curriculum. There are now specialists in oral and maxillofacial radiology (OMR), the newest dental specialty. Out of the approximately

two hundred thousand dental professionals in the United States, there are very few of these specialists, and most of them are dental school faculty. Rather than sending scans to one of these experts for review, most dentists take continuing education courses to learn how to review the scans themselves. Depending on the knowledge and experience of the individual dentist, this may or may not be sufficient.

Second, once the machine is installed, there's tremendous financial pressure to recommend its use. Ask your dentist if a CBCT scan is the best possible way to obtain the diagnostic information. Is it the least amount of radiation and the lowest cost while still fulfilling the objective? In many cases, it may be, but it doesn't hurt to confirm this. Remember—you are the best advocate of your dental health.

RADIATION

X-rays, like microwaves, are part of a spectrum and invisible to the human eye. Because we can't see X-rays, the anxiety for patients is that they may be getting too much radiation. Ionizing radiation, which includes ultraviolet light, radon, and X-rays, can cause harm by penetrating human tissue and causing cellular changes. Radon, which accounts for a sizeable portion of ionizing radiation, is the second-leading cause of lung cancer in the United States.[6]

There is even natural radioactivity—however minuscule—in food. The high level of potassium in bananas contains some radioactivity, but this doesn't mean you should avoid eating bananas. Tobacco, however, is another matter: As if there weren't enough reasons not to smoke, tobacco contains small amounts of radioactive material that settles in the lungs of smokers.

Radiation originates from background radiation and man-made sources. Background radiation is all around us, from the granite in our kitchen countertops to ultraviolet rays from the sun. The National Council on Radiation Protection and Measurements (NCRP) estimates that the average person in the United States gets 3.1 millisieverts (mSv) of background radiation per year from natural sources. If you live in high altitude, that amount is higher. Frequent air travel also results in more background radiation. Another 3.1 mSv annually comes from man-made sources, primarily X-rays, CT scans, PET scans, and nuclear medicine procedures.[7] Dental radiography accounts for only 2.5 percent of all medical radiation.[8]

Common Radiation Statistics

The purpose of the following chart is not to confuse you with numbers. Rather, it's to show you that compared to the 3.1 millisieverts of annual background radiation each of us receives, the radiation from dental X-rays is negligible.

One periapical film X-ray	0.005 mSv
One periapical digital X-ray	0.002–0.003 mSv
Four film bitewings	0.038 mSv
Four digital bitewings	0.005 mSv
Full mouth film X-rays	0.171 mSv
Full mouth digital X-rays	0.01–0.03 mSv
Panoramic X-ray	0.02 mSv
One-way air travel from Los Angeles to New York City	0.035 mSv
CBCT from a root canal	0.011–0.674 mSv
CBCT from multiple implants	0.030–1.073 mSv
Round-trip air travel from Singapore to Los Angeles	0.1 mSv
Chest X-ray	0.1 mSv
Chest CT scan	7 mSv
Mammogram	0.4 mSv
Upper GI series	6 mSv

Because millisievert is not a familiar unit of measure to most people, sometimes these statistics are explained in other ways: A chest X-ray is equivalent to about eleven days of background radiation, or slightly more radiation than round trip air travel trip from Los Angeles to New York City.

Charts that outline radiation risks are based on a person thirty years of age. If you are over eighty, your radiation risks are negligible simply because the time it takes for a tumor to develop will be longer than your lifespan. The opposite applies to younger individuals. Radiation risk is three times greater for a child under ten and twice as great for the group from ages ten to twenty.[9] It's critical to make wise decisions when taking X-rays on children.

Ways for Your Dentist to Minimize Radiation

Although you may have limited input, it's helpful to understand the choices dentists make in minimizing radiation for their patients.

- Select the most appropriate X-ray. If there's more than one type that will do the job, then it must be the one that produces the least amount of radiation with the lowest cost.
- Use digital imaging, as this substantially reduces the amount of radiation. When film X-rays are developed in a darkroom or through a stand-alone processor, the process takes eight to ten minutes. If the image doesn't turn out ideally, taking an additional X-ray adds delays to the appointment, and this factors into the decision whether to retake. With digital scans, taking another image is quick and easy. In the time it takes for your dentist to say, "Let's get a better shot," the image is already on the screen. Even though the amount of radiation per exposure is lower, one study indicated that dentists may be inclined to take more X-rays digitally because of its ease of use.[10] This eliminates one of the main advantages of digital radiography: the reduction in radiation. As the patient, be on the lookout for this perfectionist approach to retakes.
- Provide patients with a lead apron and thyroid collar. The American Association of Physicists in Medicine recently advocated for discontinuance of routine gonadal and fetal shielding, based on the fact that the radiation is tens of thousands–fold lower than the amount that will cause sterility.[11] Although this position has been supported by other medical groups, the ADA and state dental associations still recommend use of a lead apron.

The thyroid, a small organ that sits at the center of the neck near the Adam's apple, is particularly sensitive to radiation. This is especially true in children. A separate thyroid collar can be used, and many aprons come with an attached collar. For panoramic X-rays and some CBCT scans, however, the thyroid collar interferes with the X-ray beam and cannot be used.

- Maintain X-ray machines and equipment. Checking and testing the settings of the X-ray machine and the software will ensure the best product while producing the lowest amount of radiation. Digital phosphor plates degrade with repeated use and can cause phantom images that interfere with the diagnostic quality.

- Train the dental assistants. Well-trained and X-ray-licensed dental assistants can complete the process in less time with greater quality. Everyone has to learn somewhere, but speak up if you feel too many errors are being made. In addition to good technique in taking and developing X-rays, training also includes competency with the machine settings and the software to produce and store the most diagnostic images.

X-ray decisions and safety practices can ensure the highest quality image with the least number of retakes. You may be able to judge some safety practices, but others will be unknown to you. If in doubt, ask.

WHEN IT SEEMS LIKE TOO MANY X-RAYS

There may be times when you that feel an excessive number of X-rays are being taken. Many situations require a larger number of X-rays to complete the procedure successfully. To understand why you should comply, don't hesitate to ask your dentist for an explanation.

- During the root canal process, it's essential to locate every canal and reach the end of each root. Since your dentist can't see through the gums and bone, X-rays assist in determining these anatomical structures. X-rays are also used to evaluate the extent of healing and the success of the procedure, so it's customary to take a follow-up X-ray at the six-month mark.

- Multiple X-rays may be required during the placement of an implant and again several months later to determine its success.

Once the implant is ready for a crown, X-rays are necessary to check that parts used in the fabrication of the crown are properly placed. More X-rays may be needed to evaluate the fit of the crown and perhaps to distinguish any residual cement that may ultimately compromise the implant.

- During orthodontic treatment, panoramic or full mouth X-rays are sometimes taken midtreatment to check the bone level or examine the slant of the roots. Understandably, parents are nervous at the prospect of undue radiation on sensitive youthful tissue. Insist on a discussion with the orthodontist if you have concerns.

- Anytime there is uncertainty during a challenging clinical situation, an X-ray may provide much-needed clarity. For example, a root may fracture during a difficult extraction and your dentist has to access the last remaining bit. Like trying to fish out a lost key from a storm drain, direct vision is impossible. An X-ray may confirm whether the root fragment has been successfully retrieved. Or there may be a large cavity below the gum; an X-ray will show how deep the cavity is and point the way to realistic options.

The key in making decisions about X-rays is to balance the minute risks with the diagnostic benefits. Properly performed, dental X-rays are a safe and effective tool in the treatment of dental disease.

6

CONFUSION IN THE DENTAL AISLE—HELP!

Stroll down the dental aisle at your local pharmacy or grocery store and you'll be astounded by the confusing array of products. Never mind the cosmetic selections; figuring out the essentials is hard enough. Which toothpaste offers the most protection? Should you spring for an electric toothbrush? What about floss? (You're supposed to floss, right?) And when do you need a mouthwash? No wonder you may suffer from decision paralysis.

TOOTHPASTE

Do we really need toothpaste? In 2008, Americans spent $1.27 billion on toothpaste alone,[1] and that number is thought to be higher today. But did you know that good oral hygiene can be achieved without toothpaste? It is the mechanical action of rubbing the teeth that removes harmful plaque. With the principal exception of fluoride and its proven cavity reduction—and over the protests of antifluoridators—we don't need toothpaste to successfully brush our teeth. Yet we all use it, myself included.

History

Around 5000 BCE, well before toothbrushes were invented, the Egyptians used toothpaste. As the millennia passed, other cultures also used toothpaste, including the Greeks, Romans, Chinese, and Indians. Varying ingredients such as burned eggshells, pumice, crushed bones, and oyster shells were used as abrasives. Powdered charcoal and salt may have been employed as detergents. The Chinese also used ginseng and herbal mints.

More recently, toothpaste in the 1800s contained soap or chalk and were sold in powdered form. Instrumental in the promotion and marketing of toothpaste, Colgate developed a toothpaste in a jar called Crème Dentifrice in the 1850s, followed by the cheaper collapsible tube in 1911. This innovative packaging has survived to the present day. In the 1950s, Procter & Gamble began adding fluoride to its toothpaste after internal research showed a reduction in cavities. Its product, Crest, became the first brand to receive an endorsement from the American Dental Association, and sales tripled. Colgate-Palmolive soon followed suit.

Sensodyne, a toothpaste for sensitive teeth, was created in the 1960s. In 1973, GlaxoSmithKline (now known as GSK) introduced Aquafresh, the first striped toothpaste and the first brand to offer freshness as a benefit. In a joint venture with Occidental Petroleum, the makers of Arm & Hammer toothpaste added a novel ingredient: baking soda. Americans readily accepted the familiarity of baking soda—already in their refrigerators—and its deodorizing and freshening properties.

During the conspicuous consumption of the 1980s, the first whitening toothpaste, Rembrandt, was introduced. Crest and Colgate soon entered the market with their own whitening products. Colgate Total Plus Whitening toothpaste was demonstrated to not only whiten but also prevent cavities and tartar buildup, earning it an ADA seal of approval. By 2008, a staggering 68 percent of toothpaste sales consisted of such whitening toothpastes, which promised to enhance both appearance and dental health.[2]

What about natural toothpastes? The word "natural" has been seized by the advertising industry to sell every product imaginable. When it comes to toothpaste, for some people, natural means a product without fluoride, yet fluoride is a naturally occurring element. For others, a toothpaste created without any man-made ingredients, like artificial flavors or colors, qualifies as natural. Still others, in objection to cruelty to animals, want only vegan products or cruelty-free animal ingredients. There are even gluten-free natural toothpastes. Selling for as much as $10 a tube, many of these products justify their premium solely on their "natural" contents.

A discussion about natural toothpastes would not be complete without the story of Tom's of Maine. Tom and Kate Chappell moved to Maine in 1968 in search of a healthier and simpler life for their young family. Frustrated at finding artificial flavors, sweeteners, and preservatives in their personal care products, they decided to create their own. In 1970, Tom's of Maine was launched. The company introduced the first natural toothpaste—without fluoride—in the United States in 1975. In 1981 Tom's added a fluoridated option, and in 2006 the company became part of the Colgate-Palmolive Company. Some of my patients were fierce devotees to Tom's dental products and a few expressed disappointment that the company now operated under one of the very same institutions that inspired the founders' mission in the first place.

Most recently, charcoal toothpastes have become a craze. Chicly black and recommended by celebrities, these products seem to be everywhere. Even Crest has gotten into the game. But with references dating back to Hippocrates, the use of charcoal as a dental hygiene product is not new. Charcoal, made from materials such as coal, wood, and peat, is activated with gas heating. This process creates many small pores within the charcoal, making it perfect for water filters or trapping poisons in cases of overdose. Somehow this capability has been expanded to include claims of "detoxifying the mouth." Not only is the mouth full of bacteria—beneficial and harmful—but there's no scientific basis for exactly what this means. Much like natural, "detoxify" has become a marketing term. Charcoal's other claim—made by a majority of charcoal toothpastes—is that it whitens teeth. While this has some validity, there are other options, such as peroxide, that produce better results. Still other experts are concerned by the abrasiveness of charcoal. Given its high price and not-always-substantiated claims, consumers should proceed with caution.

Ingredients in Toothpaste

Just as we might use a liquid cleanser to clean our sinks or shampoo to lather our hair, we use toothpaste to clean our teeth. Over the centuries, other functions have been added. Modern consumers can find toothpaste that freshens breath, fights cavities, whitens teeth, and prevents gum disease.

Toothpaste contains both active and inactive ingredients. Active components either cleanse the teeth or improve their health. Inactive ingredients include flavorings and thickeners.

- *Therapeutic agents:* These are ingredients that improve the overall health of the teeth or gums. Fluoride strengthens enamel and reduces tooth decay. All ADA-accepted toothpastes must contain fluoride. Pyrophosphates and zinc citrate have been shown to reduce the amount of tartar buildup above the gumline (supragingival). The same effect has been less well documented for tartar below the gumline (subgingival). As any dental hygienist will tell you, tartar below the gumline is much more challenging to remove, and its lingering presence contributes to the decline in periodontal health. If you have a tendency to develop a lot of tartar, then a tartar-reducing toothpaste may lessen the tartar above the gumline and improve your ability to brush around the diminished tartar buildup. But without discernable effectiveness below the gumline, it won't reverse your gum disease.

- *Cleaning agents:* These are abrasives that assist in cleaning and removing surface stains. As recently as 1945, toothpastes contained soap—giving new meaning to the punishment of "washing your mouth out with soap"! Today's cleaning agents include calcium carbonate, magnesium carbonate, aluminum oxides, silica gels, phosphate salts, and silicates.

- *Foaming and thickening agents:* Foaming agents provide toothpaste with the feel of a good detergent. Sodium lauryl sulfate, a foaming agent also found in shampoos and laundry detergents, is the most widely used. Others include sodium cocoyl glutamate and lauryl glucoside. Thickening agents bind the toothpaste together in a stable consistency. Mineral or seaweed colloids, natural gums, and synthetic cellulose are examples of such binders.

- *Desensitizing agents:* Toothpastes such as Sensodyne contain elements such as potassium nitrate, stannous fluoride, or strontium chloride that reduce tooth sensitivity.
- *Whitening agents:* These include hydrogen peroxide, carbamide peroxide, and baking soda. Due to the limited exposure time and potency, experts question the real whitening capabilities of toothpastes; other products may be more effective to whiten teeth.
- *Flavoring agents:* Even in our toothpaste, we apparently crave sugar. Artificial sweeteners like saccharin are added to toothpaste, as well as naturally occurring substances such as xylitol and sorbitol. Mint, cinnamon, and an assortment of fruit flavors are often used.
- *Humectants:* Ingredients such as glycerol, propylene glycol, and sorbitol prevent water loss in toothpaste.

Which Toothpaste Should You Pick?

Ask a dozen dentists which toothpaste they prefer and you'll likely get twelve different answers. I happen to use Crest's cavity protection toothpaste, not gel. This is mostly out of habit, as I've grown accustomed to its taste and its powder blue color.

- Select a toothpaste that fits your needs. If you shy away from ice in your drinks or consume cold beverages only using a straw, you might consider a desensitizing toothpaste. Depending on the active ingredient, it may take several weeks for the sensitivity to diminish. To brighten your smile and remove some surface stains, pick a whitening toothpaste, but bear in mind that this may cause sensitivity in your teeth. If you develop vast amounts of tartar above the gumline, go with a tartar control brand. (In general, these people also develop a fair amount of subgingival tartar, so regular teeth cleanings are advised.)
- Check for the ADA Seal of Acceptance. In order to qualify for this ADA status, toothpaste must meet three criteria: First, the toothpaste must be safe; second, it must contain fluoride; and third, it must not contain any material that will promote tooth

decay, such as added sugar. While I may never convince the antifluoridators of the therapeutic benefits of fluoride, there must be a reason that almost every dentist recommends its use.

- Take into account possible allergens. There is a slew of ingredients that may cause irritation or, seldomly, allergic responses. The most common culprits are flavorings, predominantly mint and cinnamon. Detergents that give toothpaste its foaminess, such as sodium lauryl sulfate (SLS) or cocamidopropyl betaine (CAPB), can cause canker sores. Propylene glycol is a third offender. All can contribute to reactions like burning mouth, sores, itching, and red, cracking lips. If you experience any of these symptoms, stop using the toothpaste immediately. Study the ingredients for potential reasons, and as you would with a food allergy, utilize a systematic approach in figuring out the source of your irritation if possible. Select a toothpaste without sodium lauryl sulfate, cinnamon, or mint and see if symptoms develop.

- Read labels and recognize fads. Determine exactly what words like "natural," "organic," or "detoxifying" mean. A more expensive toothpaste in an elegantly designed package doesn't necessarily translate into a better product.

- Maybe you can forgo the toothpaste entirely. Remember—you don't really need it. You could substitute with plain brushing followed by a fluoride rinse, or even use an old, proven homemade toothpaste recipe: a slurry of peroxide, baking soda, and water.

TOOTHBRUSHES

Dating back to 3500–3000 BCE, Babylonians and Egyptians used twigs to make toothbrushes by chewing on one end until it was frayed. In addition to rudimentary toothpastes, twigs were also used to freshen breath. Many such twigs contained tannin, an astringent with antibacterial capabilities. In India, neem chewing sticks have been used to clean teeth since the fifth century BCE. With strong antimicrobial properties, neem sticks are still very popular in rural India, and they are available for purchase from Amazon and eBay.

The Chinese are credited with inventing the first natural-bristle toothbrush, which was made from pig necks. Around 1780, an imprisoned Englishman invented the first modern toothbrush. He salvaged a small animal bone, drilled holes into it, and inserted pig hair bristles. Toothbrushes with animal hair bristles were used until Dupont manufactured the first nylon bristled toothbrush in 1938. Yet it was not until after World War II that brushing gained widespread popularity among Americans. Brushing and shaving—two practices the US Army made obligatory—came home with the soldiers and gained traction with the American public.

What to Look for in a Toothbrush

Regardless of whether you use a manual or electric toothbrush, the same guidelines apply:

- Size matters. Select the tuft of bristles that easily fits into your mouth and gives you plenty of room to maneuver.
- Choose a handle that fits comfortably in your grasp. In cases of compromised manual dexterity, such as Parkinson's, a larger handle that is easier to hold is beneficial.
- Go with soft bristles only, whether it's nylon or natural. Anything stiffer may cause injury to your gums.
- Look for the ADA Seal of Acceptance.
- And remember, you don't need anything expensive, fancy, or gimmicky.

Electric Toothbrushes

Maybe your needs would be better served with an electric toothbrush. The first electric toothbrush, the Swedish Broxodent, appeared in the United States in 1960. Since then, the market for nonmanual brushes has grown worldwide.

Nonmanual brushes are either battery operated or rechargeable. In general, the battery-operated ones are cheaper and require the user to do more of the work of brushing. Like cars, electric brushes are available with many options. Or you can buy a simple one with a

built-in two-minute timer. There is pressure for brush manufacturers to introduce new and improved features every year, such as a UV
light to destroy remaining bacteria on the brush. These features add
significantly to the cost, yet the proven benefits are unclear. Avoid
paying for features you won't use.

Keep in mind that brush heads need to be replaced with the same
frequency as a manual brush. Keep a record of the manufacturer and
model number to make reordering of brush heads less confusing.
Long after the packaging has been discarded, you may discover that
the model number is absent from the brush itself. This makes identifying the correct brush head challenging. Further, finding inventory
can be difficult and involve searches of multiple online sites. Manufacturers sometimes discontinue models—and their corresponding
brush heads. If an electric brush is being advertised for an abnormally
low price, check to determine if that model will be discontinued in the
near future. You can either stock up on brush heads or purchase off-
brand but compatible heads if you choose to purchase such a brush.

One reaction that is seldom anticipated is that the electric brush
tickles. For a few, this is intolerable. Fortunately, with a change of the
brush head, the toothbrush can be gifted to another family member.
Another possibility is to convince a family member to let you try their
brush—with a new brush head—before purchasing one yourself.

There are distinct advantages to using an electric toothbrush.
Most research has shown the electric toothbrush to be more effective than a manual one at removing plaque. It's difficult to determine
how much the timer influences this improved efficacy, since manual
brushes don't come with one. Virtually all electric brushes include a
two-minute timer and emit an alert every thirty seconds to remind
you to move on to the next quadrant. To counteract overbrushing,
some brushes shut off automatically after two minutes. With a manual
brush, unless some other means is used to record brushing time,
people tend to brush less than the prescribed two minutes.

Electric brushes are now "smart." Like hearing aids, some have
Bluetooth capability and can pair to your phone. Brushing time can
be tracked using an app, much like the ones that track the number of
daily steps. Apps can also provide coaching and encouragement. They
can motivate children by treating brushing like a game, complete with

rewards. In the future, there may be sensors that tell you if you've missed a spot.

With these advantages, should you rush out and buy an electric toothbrush? It depends. You can buy a manual toothbrush for as little as a dollar, but you'll be paying twenty-five to one hundred times that for an electric model. Answer this question first: How well are you currently brushing your teeth with a manual brush? Before your next cleaning appointment, brush your teeth and then ask your dentist or hygienist to evaluate your performance. If you need to improve, consider investing in an electric brush. Alternatively, you can purchase some inexpensive disclosing tablets at your local pharmacy. Brush your teeth, then chew one of these pink tablets and swish it around your mouth. Any areas you missed while brushing will turn pink. If you notice a sea of pink, consider buying an electric brush.

There are specific groups who require more help with brushing and an electric brush will serve their needs. Children—or anyone—with metal braces should use an electric brush. People with physical impairments, even temporary ones like a broken dominant arm, would benefit. This group may include patients with conditions such as Parkinson's, arthritis of the hands, or visual impairment, as well as elderly patients with declining dexterity.

And if you happen to receive an electric toothbrush as a gift, by all means, use it.

BEST PRACTICES WITH BRUSHING

- Brush your teeth twice a day, in the morning and before bed, for two minutes. If you can do it only once, brush at night. Because saliva flow decreases substantially during sleep, the most critical time to brush your teeth is right before bedtime. Residual food and sticky plaque will not be left to fester and invite cavities.
- If you wish to go above and beyond in your oral hygiene, brush after every meal and snack, especially if you've eaten something sweet and sticky. Bear in mind, though, that many foods, especially carbohydrates and sugar, will cause the pH to drop in your mouth and create an acidic environment. Brushing under such

circumstances may actually damage the teeth. So wait half an hour after eating before you brush.

- After vomiting or acid reflux, wait a minimum of half an hour before you brush due to the acidity of stomach juices. To neutralize the acid and eliminate some of the bad taste, you can rinse your mouth with a mixture of water and baking soda instead.

- There is the danger of overbrushing, especially if you are heavy handed. You risk injuring your gums and eroding the roots of your teeth. When switching to an electric toothbrush from a manual brush, be careful not to push or use any pressure. Instead, passively hold and guide the electric brush—and allow it to do its job.

- There is no one single way to brush effectively, but a systematic approach is best. One method is to start with your upper teeth. Begin on the outside from right to left, then brush the chewing surfaces, and finish on the tongue side. Repeat the process with your lower teeth. Pay particular attention to the gumline areas.

- Brush or use a tongue scraper to clean your tongue. This reduces the bacteria that resides in the folds and crevices and helps control bad breath.

- After each use, air-dry your brush rather than storing it in an enclosed container. Be aware of aerosol contaminants that may land on your toothbrush—in other words, don't leave your brush near the toilet.

- Don't share your toothbrush. Bacteria and other microorganisms can be transmitted in saliva.

- Change your toothbrush every three to four months. Or change it more frequently if the bristles become splayed or worn. You may be brushing too hard if the bristles become prematurely worn.

- Discard the manual brush or change the electric brush head once you've recovered from an illness such as a cold or flu to prevent reinfection.

FLOSSING

Well before 1815, when a New Orleans dentist advised his patients to use a silk thread to clean in between their teeth, ancient civilizations used horsehair. In 1882, a company began manufacturing the first commercial dental floss, made from unwaxed silk. During World War II, nylon replaced silk as a floss material. Today, there are a variety of floss choices and a multitude of gadgets to aid flossing.

Floss comes in two options: waxed or unwaxed. Proponents of waxed floss point to its ease of use, while fans of unwaxed say the strands of floss separate and cover more surface area. It's your personal preference. Floss is also available in different widths: fine, regular, or wider dental tape. Some find the tape too bulky to fit comfortably in between the teeth, but others like its thick, towel-like characteristic. Floss also comes in a variety of flavors; mint and cinnamon are common. People with sensitivity to such additives may wish to stick with unflavored floss.

Dental floss, especially the waxed kind, is surprisingly strong—and versatile. In 1994, an inmate created a rope out of dental floss and managed to escape. In a pinch, I've used floss to sew on a button, tie up a plant, or temporarily as a shoelace. I've even used it to hang my kids' papier-mâché artwork. If I could only bring one oral hygiene product onto a deserted island, hands down, I would pack floss.

Proper flossing requires placing the floss perpendicular to and in between two teeth, adapting it to the sides of each tooth as far as possible below the gum—without injuring the gum—and then repeating this for all the teeth. It can be difficult and time consuming. I've witnessed many strangled fingers with cut-off circulation from holding the floss too tightly.

Many people find flossing frustrating and near impossible, resulting in the development of a wide array of flossing substitutes:

- *Toothpicks:* The ancient Egyptians fashioned toothpicks from the sharpened end of twigs. Archaeological evidence even shows grooves on the sides of teeth from zealous toothpick use. Toothpicks are still widely used today in many cultures. In some Chinese restaurants, toothpicks on the table may be as commonplace as salt and pepper shakers. Toothpicks should never be forcefully inserted between the teeth or jammed into the gums, as this can cause gum recession and tooth damage.

- *Interdental brushes and rubber tips:* Made from softer, man-made materials, interdental brushes are variations on the tooth-pick design. Some are dainty and delicate so as not to cause harm to teeth or gums. Usually larger, proxabrushes and rubber tips are meant for bigger gaps in between teeth. Caution must be exercised in not using these devices too vigorously, lest we end up like our ancestors.

- *Floss picks and plackers:* These are instruments to help you floss without having to stick both hands in your mouth. The floss pick, created in 1963, is a Y-shaped tool that holds the floss between the tips of the Y. Floss plackers are similar in concept but smaller and disposable.

- *Floss threaders and superfloss:* Patients with bridgework or braces have teeth that are connected together. Designed like a needle threader, floss threaders and superfloss utilize a stiff end to thread the floss in between teeth at the gumline.

- *Water flossers:* Water flossers shoot a stream of water to clean in between the teeth and dislodge food particles. The original Waterpik water flosser came with a separate big reservoir for water. It has been largely replaced by the water flosser of a similar design. Water flossers are also available as a wireless handheld unit that can be used in the shower.

Do I Really Need to Floss?

In 2016, in a Dietary Guidelines for Americans report, health experts cited a lack of evidence that flossing is beneficial. They removed the recommendation not only for flossing but also brushing by eliminating this sentence that was present in the 2010 guidelines: "A combined approach of reducing the amount of time sugars and starches are in the mouth, drinking fluoridated water, and brushing and flossing teeth, is the most effective way to reduce dental caries."[3] While no mention was made about the disappearance of the brushing guideline, mainstream media picked up on the flossing exclusion.

Articles began appearing with headlines like "Feeling Guilty about Not Flossing? Maybe There's No Need."[4] Patients asked whether the admonition to floss was merely hype.

It should be pointed out that the absence of scientific evidence only means there is no data to support that flossing is good for you. But that doesn't mean it isn't. Researchers want to make impactful contributions to science and design studies that will have a greater chance of funding, rather than studying the obvious, such as the benefits of taking a shower, or brushing your teeth, or washing your clothes—or—duh—flossing? To borrow a famous quote, "Absence of evidence is not evidence of absence."

Whether it's with floss or some other means, cleaning your teeth but not the area in between them would be akin to washing your body without cleaning your feet. In his book *Keep Sharp: Build a Better Brain at Any Age*, Dr. Sanjay Gupta discusses strategies to improve brain health. Besides being the chief medical correspondent for CNN, Gupta is a trained neurosurgeon. He wrote, "Flossing—and brushing—your teeth twice daily removes food debris and bacteria buildup that can ultimately lead to gum disease and increased risk of stroke. . . . Those bacteria can increase plaque buildup in the arteries, perhaps leading to clots. Hence, flossing is now a good-for-brain habit."[5]

Tips on Flossing

I didn't begin flossing until well into adulthood, several years after graduating from dental school. Now I cannot go a day without flossing my teeth. If I run out of floss during a trip, I search for a substitute—a piece of thread or maybe even a clean strand of hair.

Here are some recommendations to help you start flossing:

- Start slow. Allot only thirty seconds, maximum, per day. If the process takes you ten minutes, it is less likely you will turn it into a habit.
- Focus on a few teeth initially. You might start with your top front teeth; alternatively, if your bottom front teeth are relatively straight, you can do those instead.

- As you become more proficient, you'll be able to floss more teeth. I just timed myself, and it took thirty seconds to floss my entire mouth. This is an attainable goal for you, too.
- Your gums will bleed at the beginning. The bleeding will decrease as your flossing frequency increases.
- Your teeth may feel slightly lifted out of their sockets and your gums may be sore or itchy. Imagine if you ran a mile after years of not exercising. Most likely you would be breathing heavily and maybe experience stomach cramps. Your legs would be sore for days afterward. Don't worry: All these symptoms will disappear as you floss (or jog) more regularly.
- The best time to floss is at night before bedtime, but that may not be the ideal time for you. Pick a time that suits your schedule and lifestyle.
- Should you floss first or brush first? While there are differing opinions on this, one recent study concluded that it's better to floss first.[6] Flossing loosens food particles and bacteria from between the teeth, and brushing clears this debris away.

MOUTHWASH

As with the other products we've discussed, there is a broad selection of mouthwashes available: some over the counter, and others by prescription only. Because mouthwashes claim to do different things, it's especially important to check for the ADA Seal of Acceptance. To earn that seal, the manufacturer must provide data to show the claim is being met, as well as demonstrate the mouthwash is safe to use.

All mouthwashes should be used as an adjunct to—and not a substitute for—brushing and flossing. The alcohol content in some mouthwashes can be higher than 20 percent, providing the fresh, tingly feeling people have come to expect. Mouthwashes should be spit out and never be swallowed, as alcohol abuse and mouthwash intoxication can be a potential issue. There have been cases of alcohol poisoning solely from drinking mouthwash.

Different Mouthwashes for Different Purposes

Mouthwashes have ingredients intended to address specific concerns.

- *Freshening breath:* Perhaps the most common reason people use mouthwash is to freshen their breath. Some mouthwashes attack the volatile sulfur compounds (VSCs) created by bacteria, one of the major causes of bad breath. Therapeutic ingredients include chlorhexidine, chlorine dioxide, cetylpyridinium chloride, and essential oils. Others contain flavorings that temporarily mask mouth odor.
- *Reducing plaque and gingivitis:* The same ingredients that reduce bad breath also reduce plaque and gingivitis, which explains why these mouthwashes are advertised to address both functions. One such ingredient, chlorhexidine, is often present in prescription mouthwashes. Long-term use of chlorhexidine should be avoided because it causes staining of the teeth and dental work. It's ideal, though, as an antimicrobial after gum surgery or wisdom teeth removal.

  Be aware that any antibacterial mouthwash will destroy not only the bad bacteria but the beneficial ones as well, and disrupt the gut microbiome. Daily, long-term use of antibacterial mouthwashes should be avoided.
- *Controlling cavities:* Mouth rinses—and some gels and pastes—containing fluoride are useful for controlling cavities. Sometimes they also alleviate chronic tooth sensitivity. In the past, some of these products were available by prescription only but are now available over the counter. Before using a fluoride product, check with your dentist to ensure you're not getting too much fluoride. There are also stronger fluoride pastes containing calcium and phosphate that have the potential to remineralize and reharden small cavities. Available by prescription or through your dentist, they are used sparingly in specifically targeted areas.
- *Relieving dry mouth:* Some products—available as mouth rinses, pastes, gels, sprays, and lozenges—improve dry mouth. They contain cellulose derivatives, enzymes, or animal mucins that mimic the feel of saliva. Biotene is one popular brand. People

with dry mouth should avoid mouthwashes containing alcohol, since this tends to dry out the mouth further.

- *Whitening teeth:* Mouthwashes with either hydrogen or carbamide peroxide can whiten teeth. However, a better result may be achieved by other means such as bleaching, which allows for prolonged contact with the teeth. As with any whitening product, tooth sensitivity may be a temporary side effect.
- *Alleviating pain:* Some rinses can help to reduce pain and facilitate eating for people with mouth sores. These can occur in patients undergoing radiotherapy or chemotherapy as well as those suffering from autoimmune diseases or similarly debilitating conditions. These mouthwashes typically contain local anesthetics like topical lidocaine. Compound pharmacies can also mix specialized rinses that include a topical anesthetic, a coating agent like Maalox, an antihistamine such as Benadryl, an antifungal like Nystatin, or an antibiotic. Since these rinses must be used multiple times daily, they can be expensive. Other dentists and healthcare providers such as oncologists or cancer support groups advocate an inexpensive homemade warm water mixture of baking soda and salt.

A WORD ABOUT OIL PULLING

Oil pulling is an ancient Indian ayurvedic oral hygiene regimen that has recently become popular among natural health enthusiasts. First thing in the morning on an empty stomach, a tablespoon of oil is swished around the mouth for an entire twenty minutes. The oil disrupts bacteria and "pulls" it into the liquid, thereby removing the offending microorganisms from the mouth. When done properly, the viscous oil becomes thinner and milky white. Organic cold pressed oils from sunflower, sesame, or coconut are ideal. Coconut oil, which contains lauric acid, transforms into a soaplike substance in the presence of saliva. Olive oil can also be used. Care must be taken not to swallow or aspirate the oil into the lungs. As with cooking oil, it's best not to dump it down the drain.

Limited research indicates that oil pulling reduces the microbial count and has positive oral hygiene effects.[7] Because of its low cost and ready availability, oil pulling may be an alternative to mouthwashes. But like mouthwashes, it shouldn't be used as a substitute for brushing and flossing.

7

I WANT THAT PERFECT SMILE ON INSTAGRAM—BUT ARE THOSE FAKE TEETH?

A brief Google search on the history of cosmetic dentistry yields little beyond websites for individual dental practices selling cosmetic dentistry. Yet concern with the aesthetics of teeth dates back to the ancient Egyptians, who whitened their teeth four thousand years ago with a paste of pumice stone and wine vinegar. But it was not until the 1980s that cosmetic dentistry really grew in the United States.

Several trends converged to popularize cosmetic dentistry. The benefits of fluoride, sealants, and awareness of dental hygiene resulted in less tooth decay in patients who could afford dentistry. Dentists were less busy and became receptive to other sources of revenue. At the same time, products such as porcelains, tooth-colored resins, and bonding agents were introduced, giving dentists many more aesthetic treatment options. And in 1982, the Supreme Court lifted the long-standing restrictions against medical advertising, allowing dentists to tout their cosmetic expertise and openly compete for patients. The stage seemed set for everyone to have a Hollywood smile.

Forty years later, the bright American smile is an aspirational commodity marketed around the world. The global cosmetic dentistry market is expected to reach $35.6 billion by 2028.[1]

From simple to complex, there are many options to improve the appearance of your teeth. Follow this fundamental edict: *Do the least to achieve the most.* But as a patient, how do you even begin to determine that? It's crucial to educate yourself on the treatment possibilities. Ask questions. Seek more than one opinion.

Cosmetic dentistry is not recognized as a specialty by the American Dental Association. There is no prescribed additional training that results in another advanced degree. In short, any dentist can call themselves a cosmetic dentist, so it's unnecessary to seek out a specialist. The majority of dentists have some expertise and experience in providing this kind of treatment, but knowledge and experience can be variable among dentists. There are membership organizations such as the American Academy of Cosmetic Dentistry that provide dentists opportunities for continuing education, certification, and fellowship.

You may be thinking, "These are my front teeth and I want them to be perfect!" But before you go to an expensive dentist-to-the-stars, start with your family dentist. You have an ongoing relationship with this professional, who will provide an honest assessment—and you may be surprised to learn that she does a fair number of veneers. Trust that she'll make the right decision about whether to refer you. Asking your family dentist is also a professional courtesy; if you bypass her entirely, she may feel overlooked. Since your relationship will continue beyond this immediate cosmetic work, it's mutually beneficial to maintain rapport.

BLEACHING

Americans spend more than $1 billion a year on teeth-whitening products alone,[2] benefiting the likes of everyone from Procter & Gamble to CVS to individual dentists. There is even a store in my neighborhood devoted exclusively to walk-in "organic" teeth whitening, with two other locations in the city. Everyone, it appears, wants whiter teeth.

If you're happy with the size, shape, and alignment of your teeth and you simply want to brighten them up a bit, then you are the ideal candidate for bleaching. Most people will achieve a result of several shades lighter from bleaching, or you may require more extensive cosmetic procedures to get the smile you desire, but before you embark on that treatment, ask yourself if you're satisfied with the color of your teeth. If the answer is no, consider bleaching first.

Like any cosmetic work, bleaching is optional. Multiple times a day I would be asked, "Do you think I should bleach my teeth?" With the exception of somebody getting a new front crown (discussed in chapter 9), my response was always, "It's your decision. I can't answer that question for you." I didn't want to add to the societal pressure and emphasis on youth and beauty, but when pressed, I readily admitted to bleaching myself; I had succumbed to the marketing ploys.

Get an exam first, though. Even if you decide to bleach with an over-the-counter product, have your dentist examine your teeth first. He can rule out any underlying issues or areas that may be harmed by the bleach ingredients.

How Bleaching Works

Much like the polishing at the conclusion of a cleaning appointment or the use of a whitening toothpaste, bleaching removes extrinsic surface stains that develop from contact with foods and beverages that stain or from smoking. More importantly, it also lightens the intrinsic stains that originate from inside the tooth, which worsen with age.

The most commonly used—and most effective—bleaching agents are carbamide peroxide and hydrogen peroxide. A precursor, carbamide peroxide actually turns into hydrogen peroxide, so in effect, the two agents are nearly identical. Both are available in varying concentrations.

Limitations of Bleaching

It's important to have realistic expectations. If your teeth started out a dingy yellowish brown, no amount of bleaching will bring them to a dazzling white. An achievable goal is an improvement of several shades. Take all the dramatic before-and-after pictures with a measure of skepticism. The after pictures are usually taken at the completion of the procedure, when teeth appear their whitest due to dehydration. As moisture is incorporated back into the teeth, they will darken. Results can sometimes be unpredictable. While most teeth bleach as expected, some show very little improvement, but I have also been surprised by others that have lightened substantially and unexpectedly. Sometimes there's no explanation.

- There are some situations where no improvement will be seen even after a full bleaching regimen. One such situation is tetracycline staining, greyish-brownish coloring that can develop in people who took the antibiotic as children. In my experience, I've seen only mild improvement after months and months of bleaching. The other case is severe fluorosis. When a child ingests a higher than recommended amount of fluoride, the developing permanent teeth will be discolored in a range from yellowish to brownish. The darker the color, the less likely it will lighten.
- You will get relapse. The newly bleached color should remain stable for six to twelve months on average, but this depends on your dietary habits. If you drink red wine or dark coffee, or eat blueberries regularly, the color will darken quicker. The same goes for smoking. It likely will not relapse to its original color, though. To maintain the bleached shade, you will need to repeat the process occasionally. This usually is a more abbreviated touch-up treatment.
- Only the enamel will whiten. Crowns or veneers, which are made of artificial materials, will not chemically bleach and will remain the same color. This is especially important for people with crowns or veneers on prominent front teeth. There may be a silver lining, though. Usually crowns are lighter in color to begin with, since the rest of the teeth have darkened over the years. The roots of teeth contain cementum and are not covered by enamel. If there is recession in your mouth such that the roots are exposed, they will also not change color during the bleaching process. With a wide smile, you may show a two-tone color landscape.

- Preexisting white spots on your teeth will also lighten in color. Often they may even appear exaggerated in their whiteness. Over time, the white areas will fade and blend into the surrounding enamel. An ideal solution for this would be some kind of block-out material that can be placed over those spots prior to bleaching, but no such option currently exists.
- Resist the temptation to overbleach. I can spot overbleached teeth from afar; they take on a bluish tint, not unlike the blue ice in a glacier. Overbleaching can increase the risk of permanent harm to your teeth or dental work. Follow the manufacturer's recommendations regarding frequency of use.

Dentist-Supervised Bleaching Options

Dentist-supervised options include bleaching that occurs entirely in the dentist's office and home bleaching where the preparatory work is done by your dentist. The two methods are not mutually exclusive. Some patients start with an in-office bleaching boost and follow up with home bleaching, either to gradually improve the result or as a touch-up when needed.

In-Office Bleaching In-office bleaching is typically a one-time procedure. After your teeth have been flossed and polished to remove the superficial stains, a strong bleaching agent is applied directly to them. The entire process, which takes about an hour, is usually done by a dental assistant.

Care must be taken to protect the gums from any contact with the bleach, as even minimal contact will cause temporary injury to the gum. But no matter how much care is taken, chances are some areas will become irritated. You may feel a tingling or burning sensation, and the tissue will turn white. Any pain is typically brief, and the gum will return to its natural pink in a few hours or less. Topical vitamin E oil is a good soothing agent, squeezed directly from a hole in a vitamin E capsule.

Since its introduction, the cost of in-office bleaching has decreased due to competition from the over-the-counter marketplace. Sometimes dentists provide in-office bleaching at no charge as an incentive to begin comprehensive cosmetic treatment. If this is offered, consider accepting and bleaching your teeth before starting treatment.

Some dentists advocate a light source, a laser, or a heat source, claiming that it enhances the bleaching results. There is strong evidence to indicate that lights and lasers have no significant influence over the color outcome.[3] Additionally, a heat source may, in fact, be harmful to the nerve inside the teeth.

At-Home Bleaching Home bleaching with trays is another dentist-supervised method. With this option, impressions are taken at the dentist's office from which thin custom trays are fabricated. The trays are then used as a reservoir for the bleaching agent. As the name implies, you do the bleaching yourself at home, usually over the course of a couple weeks.

When this procedure was introduced, patients were encouraged to leave the trays on overnight. While this is still one option, now most people wear the trays for an hour or so. In general, the bleaching agent used for the home bleaching technique is weaker than the in-office variety.

If you already have trays, check them to see if they're scalloped. Initially, trays were made to cover over part of the gum. This meant the gums were coming into contact with the bleach unnecessarily. A scalloped tray that follows the contours of your teeth and ends where the tooth and gum meet is preferable. Trays can be easily and quickly adapted to create this shape.

Do-It-Yourself Bleaching Options

I had one patient who took do-it-yourself to new heights. He soaked some cotton in hydrogen peroxide, placed it over his teeth, and then wrapped the cotton with Saran Wrap. But for almost everyone else, the do-it-yourself method usually involves the purchase of over-the-counter products.

Toothpastes promise to whiten. So do mouthwashes. There are paint-on gels and even whitening chewing gum. Then there's the familiar Crest Whitestrips. It's all so confusing—which product is right for you? A recent review of over-the-counter bleaching research revealed a winner: Whitestrips showed superior efficacy compared to all other over-the-counter products.[4] Whitening toothpastes placed a distant second in that they removed extrinsic stains only.

Tooth Sensitivity

When bleaching was first introduced, practically every patient suffered from the side effect of tooth sensitivity. Since then, ingredients such as amorphous calcium phosphate (ACP) have been added to some products to reduce sensitivity. In general, the higher the concentration of the bleaching agent, the greater the likelihood of sensitivity. There is a lot of individual variability, though. For a rare few, bleaching is impossible because their teeth become ultrasensitive to the point of being intolerable. The sensitivity is temporary, though, and over time, it dissipates.

There are strategies to reduce sensitivity:

- Several weeks before bleaching, use a toothpaste that reduces tooth sensitivity, such as Sensodyne, on a daily basis. Continue using this throughout the process.
- If that's not sufficient, ask your dentist about an ACP relief gel that can be dispensed inside your bleaching tray. This can either be done concurrently when bleaching or separately.
- Consider reducing the concentration of the bleaching agent. Many studies have shown that using a weaker agent for a longer period of time actually produces better results. Reduce the frequency of the bleaching, either by doing it every other day or shortening the prescribed time.

RECONTOURING

Recontouring—or enameloplasty—is the slight shaping of teeth. Minor adjustments can make a tremendous impact in a tooth's appearance and its overall appearance relative to the rest of the teeth. This is a quick, simple, and inexpensive method of improving your smile.

It is also underutilized. One of the main reasons is that there's no insurance billing code associated with enameloplasty, leaving dentists confused about how much to charge for this simple procedure.

There are no hard-and-fast rules as to when enameloplasty is appropriate, but obvious cases present themselves. Perhaps recontouring is best explained using examples:

- Over the years, the edges of your front teeth have turned jagged: a chip here and there, perhaps with some areas that look like you've used your teeth to open bottles. The teeth are still fairly long, though. Leveling off the edges and reshaping them will not result in out-of-proportion teeth. In fifteen minutes, you'll have a polished new look.
- One tooth is hanging down below your other teeth, drawing the eye to the disharmony. Provided there's enough enamel and no sensitivity, that single tooth can be adjusted to match its neighbors. I did this with one of my own teeth, a lower front one that was sticking up.
- Teeth that are square and angular in shape connote a masculine impression, whereas rounded teeth suggest a softer feminine appearance. A subtle rounding of certain corners of square teeth can dramatically alter appearance.

Because recontouring involves only the enamel—which has no nerve endings—no pain is felt and no anesthetic is necessary. In fact, anesthetic is discouraged. Your dentist will need input, though, if she's getting close to the dentin layer, where sensation can be felt. Recontouring does involve some loss of your tooth's finite enamel, but it is still a lot more conservative than any other cosmetic procedure.

Not every dentist will offer enameloplasty as a solution. Some may not be able to visualize it. Still others may recommend more extensive—and expensive—options.

BONDING

While recontouring is subtractive, bonding is additive. Bonding assumes the underlying tooth is healthy. If the tooth has a large cavity or is structurally unsound—and needs cosmetic improvement—then a different procedure such as a veneer or crown may be indicated.

Bonding involves using composite resin—the same material ubiquitously used in white fillings—to fill in gaps or cover over teeth to improve their shape and appearance. The term "bonding" is derived from the process: The composite resin is chemically bonded onto the tooth. Composite resins have come a long way. My early experience using composites was nerve-racking. It came in two containers from which equal parts were dispensed. Once the mixing began, the clock started ticking, and I rushed to complete the procedure before the composite hardened into a stubborn lump. Today, dentists can place the composite meticulously and leisurely; when satisfied, they turn on an ultraviolet light to harden the material. What used to be a single color choice is now a wide variety of shades, giving dentists the ability to create a perfect color match. Moreover, the characteristics of the material have improved in terms of durability, strength, and aesthetics. With bonding, your dentist can create a realistic, lifelike tooth in a single appointment.

To do this, the dentist must be an artist. Excellent bonding is difficult to master and very technique sensitive. It helps if your dentist has a painter's eye for color and can select just the right mix of pigmentation to match your other teeth. Color can look different in different lights, though. Your tooth may be indistinguishable in sunlight yet stand out under fluorescent lighting. Bonding often entails trial and error—and patience on the part of your dentist. And this is why your dentist may not offer bonding as a first choice. It's much more challenging to match one chipped front tooth than it is to replace both front teeth with a uniform color in a more expensive procedure. Your dentist may conclude—perhaps justifiably so—that he doesn't get paid enough for the effort and time it takes to match a single tooth, or maybe he's not confident in his artist's eye.

But what if bonding is the best choice? Maybe bonding is the most conservative option, one that preserves the bulk of your own teeth.

Have an honest discussion with your dentist regarding the pros and cons of each path.

Ideal Situations for Bonding

- *Small gaps in between front teeth:* Gaps between the upper front teeth, known as diastemas, are notoriously challenging to keep closed, even after braces. African Americans are more predisposed to exhibit such spaces. Depending on the width of the diastema, bonding can offer the ideal treatment.
- *Multiple small gaps:* Sometimes the teeth adjacent to the upper front teeth (lateral incisors) are genetically abnormally small. Again, depending on the width of the spaces, bonding may be a good option, either on the lateral incisors alone or in combination with the other front teeth.
- *The chipped tooth:* Bonding is the ideal solution if a small corner of a front tooth breaks off. A drawback is that the material may not stay on for a prolonged period of time. But even if the procedure must be repeated occasionally, this is still the most conservative option.
- *The hidden tooth:* Occasionally the teeth are too large for the jaw and one tooth gets squeezed out of position, leaving it behind the round arc formed by the other teeth. The front of the hidden tooth can be bonded to fool the eye, bringing it into alignment with its neighbors without actually moving the tooth.
- *Almost anything involving the lower front teeth:* By nature, the lower incisors are small, dainty objects, and procedures such as crowns may present risky complications. Sometimes crowns are the only alternative, but bonding should be considered as a more conservative option when possible.

Advantages and Disadvantages

On the positive side, bonding is reversible! You may finally close the diastema between your upper front teeth and subsequently decide it changes your entire face. You don't recognize yourself. The bonding can be carefully removed to return your teeth to their original condition. Bonding is conservative, since very little, if any, of the tooth is drilled away. Because there's no invasive drilling, no anesthetic is required.

One disadvantage of bonding is that as a material, composite resin doesn't hold up as well over time. Depending on your habits, composite can stain, especially if the surface hasn't been polished adequately. It can also chip or fall out. However, with today's excellent bonding agents, the composite has a much greater likelihood of remaining secure.

And, as noted earlier, dentist skill factors into bonding more so than most procedures.

VENEERS

That celebrity with the gleaming, perfect smile—the one you want—probably has a mouthful of veneers. A veneer is a thin shell, made of porcelain or a similar material, that is bonded onto the outer surface of a relatively healthy and cavity-free tooth. A veneer can change the color and shape of the underlying tooth, but not its orientation. If the alignment of the teeth is the issue, consider orthodontic treatment first. While a single veneer can be done, in general, veneers are planned for groups of teeth.

Veneers generally require two appointments spaced one to three weeks apart. Anesthetic, drilling, impressions, some kind of temporary fabrication, and possibly photos occur during the first visit. The veneers are delivered at the second appointment, followed by more photos.

Some Considerations

Before you commit to veneers, ask your dentist if bonding would achieve the same result. Aside from being reversible, bonding is substantially cheaper than veneers and also less time consuming for both patient and dentist.

- Veneers are technique sensitive. Ask your dentist about her experience. How many veneers does she usually do annually? Ask to see before-and-after photos of her work. Presumably you have an ongoing relationship with this dentist, so don't be afraid to ask whether she's comfortable and confident treating you in this capacity or if she'd rather refer you to someone else.

- Does your dentist have a solid working relationship with an excellent lab technician? This is the person who will actually be making your veneers. (Some dentists have machines that can make veneers in the office, but the use of an outside lab technician is more common.)

- For both patients and dentists, planning is essential if approximately six or more veneers are being done. Start by studying photos of teeth. Do you want them to be perfectly symmetrical, or would you welcome an imperfection here and there for a more natural appearance? What shape are you envisioning—square and blunt, or more ovoid and rounded? Bring your pictures to the consultation.

- Your dentist can fabricate temporaries to match your desired final outcome. The temporaries, made from composite resin, can be tweaked until you're satisfied. Only then should the final veneers be made—as an exact duplicate of your temporaries. Because it's impossible for two people to have identical mental images, physically assessing and discussing your temporaries is critical. Not every dentist will go to such lengths, however. If you are having a mouthful of veneers done, find a dentist who will be thorough.

- Be prepared for the cost. One of the main reasons you're considering veneers is likely that you wish to change the color of your teeth. Face a mirror and smile broadly. Then count each visible tooth. That's how many veneers you'll need. Fees for veneers can range widely. On the high end, it can approach $2,500 per tooth, but you can expect to pay a minimum of $1,000–$1,500 for each tooth. Do the math and you'll find the investment can be significant.

- Veneers need to be completed in their entirety at the same time, rather than in piecemeal fashion. After all, you don't want to walk around with a two-toned smile. Ideally, all the visible teeth in one arch should be done simultaneously so the color lot is identical.

- Think carefully about color and how white you want your ve-neers. Have you ever come across a seventy-year-old man with jet-black hair or perfectly white teeth? It can present an un-natural and jarring impression. Most dentists report that patients tend to choose a whiter shade than the dentist recommends. One of my patients said, "I'm paying, so I decide," when I suggested she opt for a shade or two yellower. It is, of course, the patient's choice. Just remember the adage "Less is more."
- Listen to your dentist when he recommends you wear a night guard during sleep. Although a porcelain veneer is strengthened when bonded onto a tooth, since porcelain is a ceramic, there is always the risk of chipping and breakage. This appliance will protect your considerable investment.

SOME FINAL TIPS

- Improvement of your smile will often involve a combination of procedures. A couple teeth may simply need bleaching and slight recontouring. Teeth that have existing large fillings or large cavi-ties may require crowns. Still others will benefit from veneers or even implants. Thoughtful analysis and planning by your dentist are important.
- Sometimes the teeth are so misaligned that a "quick fix" with cosmetic procedures will only make matters worse. Your dentist may suggest orthodontic treatment prior to the cosmetic work. While it may seem unfathomable that you commit to braces or Invisalign when all you wanted was a prettier smile, in the long run, it may be necessary to achieve the best result. It's important to keep an open mind.
- Sometimes gum surgery is necessary first. Patients routinely ask to correct their "gummy smile" because they're dissatisfied with the excess display of gums. One remedy is the use of Botox, in-jected into the upper lip area to relax it and reduce the amount of visible gum. But depending on the underlying cause—which can range from a taller-than-average upper jaw to unusually

small teeth—gum surgery may be indicated prior to any cosmetic procedure.

- Your dental needs and health come first. You should always take care of any infections, cavities, or gum conditions before starting the cosmetic work. For example, if you're missing a lot of back teeth and don't have a solid bite, this will put unnecessary strain on your front teeth. Your beautiful veneers will be at risk of chipping, fracturing, or coming loose.

- Don't count on your insurance to help you cover the costs of treatment, as most cosmetic procedures will not be covered. Further, most of it will need to be done in unison. If the work needs to be sequenced for financial reasons, discuss this with your dentist and come up with a plan. X-rays, exams, repairing of a chipped tooth, night guards, and other procedures may be covered depending on your insurance plan.

- Unless you are only having your teeth bleached or the treatment involves only one tooth, you need a plan. You wouldn't embark on a remodel without a plan; the same goes for your mouth. Watch out for the dentist who talks about a "smile makeover" before addressing the health and condition of your mouth, or the dentist who is critical of the yellowness of your teeth and says you must bleach them. Beware the dentist who wants to start immediately—today—on an extensive cosmetic treatment without discussing expectations or a plan.

- As with all cosmetic procedures, it's important to ask yourself why you're doing this. Like many others, you may simply want whiter teeth and a more attractive smile. Maybe you've lived with dark tetracycline staining for far too long and you're looking forward to smiling confidently. But if your underlying expectations cannot be met by a set of veneers and involves deeper emotional or psychological elements, then that's a warning sign for you to reconsider.

And remember: *Do the least to achieve the most.*

FREQUENTLY ASKED QUESTIONS

Should I do bleaching in my dentist's office or go with the trays?

If you're not the type of person who can commit to a regimen for two weeks, then in-office bleaching is the perfect choice. If you like being able to control how white your teeth get, then the tray option will suit your needs. Plus, you'll have the added benefit of being able to touch up in the future without paying for a new procedure.

Maybe you're on a tight time schedule and your wedding is coming up in ten days. The in-office bleaching will be the best option.

Why do I have to pay so much more to have professional bleaching done?

Regardless of the technique or product, the bleaching agents—hydrogen peroxide and carbamide peroxide—are the same. The only difference is the concentration. You already know that whitening strips work. If cost is a factor, go with the over-the-counter whitening strips, but remember that the process may take a bit longer.

I'm seven months pregnant and thinking about bleaching my teeth. Is this safe?

According to the ADA, discretionary treatments such as teeth whitening should be avoided until after pregnancy and nursing. While the procedures may be safe, there's no need to take unnecessary risks.

I got hit playing basketball years ago and had to have a root canal. I noticed recently the tooth is now darker than my other teeth. What can I do?

An unrelated bleaching technique is the internal bleaching of a nonvital tooth that has had a root canal. Through a series of appointments—as many as three to five—a bleaching agent and heat are used to lighten the tooth. In this case, since the tooth is "dead," with no nerve, heat damage becomes a moot point. The color difference may be dramatic—and more than the typical improvement of several shades.

I don't really want cosmetic treatment. Can't I just live with my imperfect teeth?

Any cosmetic treatment is discretionary and totally your decision. The actress and model Lauren Hutton is famously known for the small gap between her upper front teeth (central incisors). When she was launching her career, she used mortician's wax and a butter knife to close the gap. But she was hesitant to do anything permanent, and over time, the gap became her trademark. Eventually she got a removable prosthesis for the gap that she can insert when she wishes.

Before I commit to the bonding, is there any way the dentist can help me to visualize what it will look like?

Dentists can easily add composite resin to a tooth without using the bonding agent, which adheres the material permanently to the tooth. This is an ideal way to show you the final result. Keep in mind that the composite will most likely be small, thin, and fragile and can easily break. But while it's in your mouth, take a picture.

It takes time to do these mock-ups, for which the dentist will not be compensated. Remember this when you are quoted the fee for the bonding.

I really want to do veneers but I hate the idea of drilling into my perfectly healthy front teeth, no matter how little it is. Are there any other options?

I've encountered many patients who objected to even the smallest amount of drilling, insisting they wanted to preserve their enamel. One company cleverly picked up on this, came up with a superthin no-drill veneer called Lumineers, and marketed the product directly to the consumer. A very thin veneer may not be adequate to cover the yellower color of the underlying tooth. And as thin as the veneer is, adding this extra layer can make the teeth bulky and unnatural looking. A trained eye will immediately spot that you've had a bunch of veneers placed.

8

MY DENTIST SAYS I HAVE A CAVITY . . . BUT IT DOESN'T HURT OR BOTHER ME

Most of us would be aghast at walking around without a front tooth, but for some, it's a nonissue. I once had a patient whose front tooth fell out while she was on vacation overseas. We decided that once she returned home I'd do an implant. However, by then, she had become so accustomed to the gap and saw no need for a temporary tooth during the several months it would take for the implant to heal. She confided that she liked the sideways glances she received and the incongruity of a well-groomed middle-aged woman with a hole in her mouth.

So, often when patients say, "It doesn't bother me," they mean either they don't care how something looks or they are not experiencing pain.

Provided there are no health risks, any dentist should respect the patient's wishes to not repair what may primarily be a cosmetic issue. Pain, however, deserves a closer appraisal because pain—or lack of pain—is not a reliable indicator of a problem. Whether a problem actually exists, most patients will seek treatment when something hurts. The reverse is not true: Just because something doesn't hurt does not mean there isn't a problem. Pain, it turns out, is complex and individualized.

PAIN

When you touch a hot stove, the sensation of pain is transmitted via nerve fibers (nociceptors) from your hand to the spinal cord, then to different centers in your brain. Along the way, sensation can be modulated by chemicals your body secretes to either increase or reduce the sensation of pain. For example, soldiers who suffer severe wartime injuries—ones that *should* be extremely painful—often report feeling no pain.

There are two major groups of nociceptors: A-delta fibers and C fibers. A-delta fibers are responsible for the acute, well-localized sharp and fast pain, such as from touching a hot surface. The smaller C fibers produce a poorly localized, slow chronic pain.

Referred pain occurs when the area that hurts is not the culprit responsible for the pain. A classic example is the arm and jaw pain associated with a heart attack. In the mouth, referred pain can be common. Many teeth share the same nerve, and distinguishing the offending tooth can prove confusing. Sometimes, as in the case of trigeminal neuralgia, a neurological condition characterized by intense, debilitating pain, despite the patient's insistence, the originating source of pain is not from a tooth at all.

As a subject, pain is extremely difficult to study. Its mechanism is complex, individualized, and subjective, as every person experiences pain differently. The sensation of pain is influenced by a host of factors, including psychological elements and past individual history. This may explain why a rare few dental patients actually refuse anesthetic, whereas others are hypersensitive and request numbing for a simple cleaning.

Pain can be an unreliable indicator of a dental issue that requires attention. Let's say you've just had a tooth extracted. Afterward, despite being told you might feel discomfort, you feel nothing; it's as if the procedure never happened. You conclude the dentist did a fabulous job. Or imagine you had a filling replaced, and three weeks later, the tooth still hurts and you cannot chew on that side. You've been back to the dentist, who insists the filling looks fine, but you know better. You decide he must've done something wrong.

While both of these scenarios may be true, the logic of the conclusions is faulty. Patients have very few parameters to judge treatment, and unfortunately, pain is one of them. However, pain—or lack thereof is not a reliable indicator of a job well done, nor does the absence of pain mean there's not a problem brewing.

What Pain Will Not Tell You

While pain will signal to you immediately that you have a paper cut, it will not tell you about your high blood pressure, your borderline diabetes, or your small developing cavity. Unlike the acute *ouch* of the paper cut, these chronic conditions fester gradually and quietly. Only when your blood pressure spikes uncontrollably might you experience headaches. Neuropathy in the form of numbness, tingling, or pain may ensue in your fingers and toes in the later stages of diabetes. If your cavity gets large enough, you may suffer excruciating pain.

Most conditions in the mouth are chronic. Besides tooth decay, many unhealthy situations in your mouth will not bother you until the later stages. These include gum disease, long-term infections, faulty or deteriorating dental work (restorations), cracked teeth, erupting wisdom teeth, and consequences of severely crowded teeth or sleep apnea. (Some of these topics will be discussed in later chapters.)

CAVITIES

Perhaps the most commonly heard pronouncement from your dentist is, "You have a cavity." But what is a cavity?

A tooth is divided into two parts: the crown and the roots. The visible crown is protected by an outer layer of enamel, the hardest substance in your body. Underneath the enamel is the dentin, a softer, yellowish section with nerve endings. In the center is the pulp of the tooth, which contains nerve fibers, blood vessels, and tissue.

The mostly invisible root, or roots, have no enamel; they are made of cementum, a substance similar to dentin. Inside the root is the continuation of the pulp, which narrows into a canal system that travels the length of the tooth.

Simply put, cavities—or caries—are holes in your teeth. Cavities can develop either on the crown of the tooth or on the visible root portion. When you eat or drink foods that contain sugar, bacteria—primarily *Streptococcus mutans* and *Lactobacilli*—consume the fermentable carbohydrates to produce acid. The pH in your mouth drops, and this more acidic environment causes deminer-alization—or softening—of your teeth, making it a very easy environ-ment for a cavity to start. Once formed, the hole will usually grow over time. Moderate cavities are often sensitive to cold or sugary stimuli. If the cavity becomes large enough to reach the pulp, pain and infection typically follow.

You may be wondering why some people get more cavities than others. While sugar is the essential ingredient, the likelihood of de-veloping cavities is influenced by many factors. Genetics plays a role. For instance, some people are born with softer, more porous enamel that's more prone to decay. Fluoride, either consumed or glazed onto the teeth via toothpaste, gel, or rinse, will strengthen enamel and make the teeth more resistant to cavities. Hygiene is also important in keeping cavities from forming, as is saliva, which lubricates and cleanses the mouth. Patients with dry mouths are very susceptible to tooth decay. Lastly, there's diet. Without sugar and the sugar-bacteria interaction, cavities would not be so commonplace. It would be sim-plistic to say that cavities could be prevented if we stopped eating sugar, because sugar, it seems, is everywhere.

Sugar

A nontechnical term, the word "sugar" actually refers to all types of carbohydrates. It includes the sucrose found in candy, the glucose in pasta, and the fructose in fruit. All sugars are capable of causing cavi-ties; however, sucrose is more potent than others.

Sugar used to be a luxury product. In George Washington's time, the average American consumed 6 pounds of sugar a year. By 2004, that number had jumped to 100 pounds. Today the per capita con-sumption of sugar is a stunning 150 pounds, much of it in the form of high fructose corn syrup, hidden added sugar, and cheap sweetened sodas.[1] Besides cavities, this has led to a host of health ailments, including obesity, type 2 diabetes, liver damage, and cardiovascular disease.

Even though sugar is harmful to our teeth, not all sugars are harmful to our bodies. When we *eat* an apple, the naturally occurring sugar and fiber in the fruit are absorbed slowly by the body and provide an even and useful source of energy for our bodies. However, when we *drink* a supersized soda, the sugar hits the body all at once, and our organs are incapable of metabolizing this sugar rush. When this excess sugar is converted into fat, we gain weight. Similar to drugs, we become physically addicted and crave even more sugar. And it is making us sick.

Unlike salt or trans fat, there are no federal limits on sugar. The American Heart Association recommends a daily maximum of six teaspoons (25 grams) of added sugar for women and nine teaspoons (36 grams) for men. Most people consume quite a bit more, but it would be impossible—and dreary—to avoid sugar altogether. The key is moderation.

There are several habits you can adopt to control the amount of sugar in your diet:

- Read labels. Check for hidden and added sugars in foods. We all know there's sugar in candy, but there's an astounding 13 grams of sugar in my favorite yogurt. Canned sauces are another surprising source.
- Pay extra attention to low-fat products. Low fat almost always means high sugar. In order to taste good, a low-fat product must make up for this deficit in another way. Check the sugar content of a low-fat cookie versus a traditional one.
- Avoid sugary drinks. A 16-ounce bottle of Coke contains 39 grams of sugar. Besides sodas, there are added sugars in sports drinks, teas, coffees, and other beverages.
- Eat—don't drink—your fruits. When you eat an orange, the fiber will offset the negative effects of the sugar by making it slower to absorb. When you drink a glass of orange juice, no such protection is offered. The same goes for those "healthy" smoothies, even ones made with pulverized vegetables with the fiber removed.

How to Minimize Cavities

- Avoid sticky, sugary treats. Since added sugar is a fact of life in modern diets, it's important to do what you can to minimize its effects. The stickier the sugar, the worse it is, including raisins, honey, and Fruit Roll-Ups. If you must eat these foods, try to brush your teeth afterward. However, since your mouth will be very acidic after consuming them, wait at least thirty minutes for the pH to neutralize before you brush.
- Reduce the frequency of your intake. Every time you consume something sweet, the combination of sugar and bacteria will create an acidic environment for approximately twenty minutes. It's preferable to eat those five pieces of candy all at once rather than one every hour.
- Brush your teeth before bedtime. Bedtime is the most critical time of day to ensure a clean mouth. During sleep, saliva flow virtually ceases and food residue is left to fester for hours in the crevices of your teeth. Brushing your teeth before bedtime eliminates that residue and reduces the risk of developing cavities.
- Practice good dental hygiene. In addition to watching your sugar intake, proper brushing with a fluoridated toothpaste and flossing will maintain a clean mouth. Cavity-prone individuals should consider a fluoride gel or rinse.

How Dentists Diagnose Cavities

Some cavities are visible to the naked eye. You might even be able to identify one yourself. Others can be seen on an X-ray. Tactile examination is another way to find them: When your dentist pokes at your teeth with a sharp instrument, a soft area often indicates a cavity.

Over the last twenty years, high-tech devices have become more frequently used in the hunt for cavities. Some of these devices use fluorescent lasers or infrared light to detect cavities. Others analyze the tooth's crystalline structure. Still others use algorithms to highlight vulnerable areas where cavities may develop. While false positives have been an issue, these devices can identify tiny early stage cavities. Some can even quantify the severity of a lesion. With actual numbers, progress and growth of the cavity can be objectively measured over time.

These devices serve as an adjunct to aid diagnosis. No dentist should rely on them exclusively to decide treatment.

Should Every Cavity Be Treated?

Cavities can remain the same size for years or even decades—or they can grow. It's not always easy to predict. In general, small cavities can remain stable for a long time and, as such, may not require filling.

A cavity that is confined to the enamel portion of the tooth can sometimes be reversed with fluoride remineralization products, which can help repair the enamel. But once the cavity has penetrated the dentin layer, the chances for remineralization are slim and growth is usually quicker.

Despite meticulous brushing and flossing, one of my children is cavity prone. She has a couple cavities that haven't grown in at least eight years. Her new dentist wanted to fill one of them. While his plan appeared reasonable, I advised her to take a more cautious approach and leave it alone. I did so because of my familiarity with her dental history and her fastidious dental hygiene.

Your dentist should use his judgement and experience when deciding whether to treat a cavity. He must take into account your hygiene, the cavity's age, and its progression (through analysis of previous X-rays or recordings). Bear in mind, though, that our current healthcare system rewards dentists for procedures performed rather than watchful observation. And what happens if the cavity grows unpredictably in the next six months—will you then blame him for not acting soon enough?

FAULTY RESTORATIONS

Nothing lasts forever—and that includes the dental work in your mouth. With the demands of chewing and the acidic environment in the mouth, even the best dental work will eventually show signs of wear. Some dental materials wear better than others. Silver amalgam, for example, lasts much longer than composite fillings. Porcelain and the newer tooth-colored materials may chip or crack. And although it isn't used much today, gold has the greatest longevity.

Your dentist will almost always see this deterioration long before the tooth bothers you. Listen to her. Ask to see a picture so you can understand what's happening. Try not to ignore the problem, even if you're not feeling any sensitivity or pain.

The breakdown usually begins at the junction between the tooth and the filling or crown. A small gap will develop, allowing saliva and bacteria inside the tooth. A cavity—termed "recurrent decay"—may form as a result of this opening next to—or, worse yet, underneath—the restoration. Recurrent decay can be difficult to diagnose, especially if it's lurking inside a crown, because neither an X-ray nor a visual exam will reveal the problem. I've seen whole teeth disintegrate inside a crown, essentially turning the tooth into mush. At that point, extraction is the only option.

A new restoration—filling or crown—can be done to eliminate the recurrent decay. Any new restoration, though, will be bigger than the original and encompass more of the tooth. Another option is to repair the filling or crown rather than replacing the entire restoration. It's a more conservative and less costly approach. While repairing isn't always an option, in certain cases, it may be the best option.

STRUCTURAL CRACKS IN TEETH

A crack is a splitting of part of the tooth. A crack may be shallow or deep enough to completely sever a portion of the tooth. In general, vertical cracks, which run parallel to the long axis of the tooth, are more dangerous since they are not as easily fixable as horizontal ones. Certain teeth—namely, the lower second molars and the upper premolars—are more vulnerable to cracking. This has to do with their location within the mouth and the anatomical design of the teeth. Habits like clenching—the forceful gritting together of upper and lower teeth—increase the likelihood of crack formation.

A patient might say, "It doesn't happen every time, but when I bite down, it hurts like hell. Then it disappears as quickly as it started."

When I heard this, I knew the patient had a cracked tooth. Determining which one was harder: Even with this common symptom, cracks are notoriously tough to diagnose. Three-dimensional X-ray scans and fluorescent light lasers can sometimes assist with this investigation. Most dentists will want to reproduce the symptom before proceeding with treatment to ensure they are working on the correct tooth.

Once symptoms occur and can be precisely identified to the offending tooth, a crown—which acts to brace the tooth together—is usually installed. If symptoms persist after that, a root canal may be recommended. Despite all this treatment, the prognosis remains guarded. Either the patient lives with the discomfort or, if it becomes severe, the tooth is extracted.

If a crack is discovered incidentally during an exam, even if you have no symptoms, listen to your dentist when she recommends a crown. If you feel the slightest twinge, even if it's only once a month, have the crown done right away. This will increase the likelihood that the crack will not progress further.

WISDOM TEETH

Wisdom teeth are the most common congenitally missing teeth. They are also the last to erupt, usually between the ages of sixteen and twenty-five. One in each back corner, the four teeth are actually a third set of molars.

Human jaws have changed over the millennia since our days as nomadic hunter-gatherers. One theory is that when we transitioned into farming, humans began to eat softer foods. As a result, our jaws shrank in size. With inadequate space to erupt in the modern human jaw, wisdom teeth may be evolving out of existence. But for now, the question remains: Should wisdom teeth be routinely extracted?

When I mentioned that the summer before college would be the perfect time for his son to get his wisdom teeth removed, a father laughed and said, "I'm Eastern European. We just don't do this where I come from."

In many parts of the globe, it isn't customary to routinely pull wisdom teeth. Even in developed countries where the practice is common, policies are being reevaluated. In 1998, the United Kingdom began to discourage the routine extraction of wisdom teeth. Except in cases where symptoms or pathology present, the Royal College of Physicians in Edinburgh echoes this advice.[2] In the United States and Australia, removal of impacted wisdom teeth—those wholly or partially buried under the gum—is still considered standard procedure. Americans spend an estimated $3 billion a year on wisdom teeth removal.[3]

But is the routine removal of wisdom teeth warranted? The thinking goes like this: There is, and will continue to be, insufficient room in your mouth for the third molars. To prevent any future adverse effects, the wisdom teeth should be extracted prophylactically. Surgery and healing become more difficult as we age, so removal later in the event of a problem could be more challenging.

Proponents of removal cite the challenge of keeping this area clean, leading to possible tooth decay and gum infections. There's also the potential of cyst or tumor formation around the wisdom tooth. Lastly, extraction is easier before the roots are fully formed.

Perhaps the most common reason to advocate for removal is that the wisdom teeth will push and crowd your other teeth, specifically the lower front ones. Research indicates that this simply is not true. In a scientific literature review, it was found that "83 percent of articles did not find any significant relationship between lower third molar and mandibular dental anterior crowding."[4] But this myth has been repeated so many times that patients—and even dentists—believe it.

Regardless of the presence of the third molars, teeth have a natural tendency to migrate toward the center of the mouth over time. This is particularly evident with the lower front area. Look at the mouths of seniors and you'll find most have crowded lower front teeth.

There's not enough concrete evidence to recommend the wholesale extraction of wisdom teeth. Fully erupted functional third molars should be treated like any other molar. Impacted wisdom teeth should be monitored individually. Often, one problematic wisdom tooth can be extracted while leaving the other three intact.

Further, as with any surgical procedure, there are associated risks. Complications include infection, uncontrolled bleeding, and, rarely, nerve damage and allergic reactions. Modern three-dimensional X-ray scanning will accurately show the location of the nerve in relation to the wisdom tooth and aid the surgeon in substantially reducing any nerve damage.

Research is currently underway to explore the possibility of using microwave ablation, also called microablation, to disintegrate wisdom teeth.[5] This nonsurgical technique is commonly used to treat tumors and may provide a less invasive approach.

So When Should You Get a Wisdom Tooth Removed?

- *Repeated infection or pain:* Third molar infections (pericoronitis) are often accompanied by pain, swelling, and an inability to open your mouth fully or chew normally. They're also not isolated incidents and can recur. If you suffer from repeated bouts of pericoronitis, extract the tooth.
- *Decay:* Cavities can occur either in the wisdom tooth or the preceding one (second molar). If a cavity develops in the second molar and treatment becomes difficult because the wisdom tooth is in the way, then removal is indicated. Depending on the extent and location of a cavity in an impacted wisdom tooth, it can be either filled or extracted. Barring complicating factors, a fully erupted third molar should be preserved and filled.
- *Gum problems:* Sometimes the orientation of the wisdom tooth will create gum problems in the second molar. To prevent compromising the second molar, remove the wisdom tooth.
- *Cyst formation:* Any suspicious X-ray that hints at the presence of a cyst or tumor is grounds for removal of the wisdom tooth.
- *Unusual soft tissue changes:* The partially erupted wisdom tooth may be causing you to constantly bite your cheek, turning it red and raw. Or an upper wisdom tooth without a corresponding lower one will grow until it touches the lower gum. As it persistently presses on the gum, it will turn the tissue white. Both these situations warrant removal of the tooth.
- *Before braces:* Braces are usually undertaken to correct crowded teeth. Where there is room, teeth will be moved toward the back

of the mouth to straighten them. If that space is occupied by wisdom teeth, they should all be extracted.

- *To prevent radionecrosis or osteonecrosis:* In rare instances, radiation therapy or intravenous osteoporosis medication can cause spontaneous destruction of portions of jawbone. Although not entirely understood, necrosis is related to an inadequate blood supply. Prior to such procedures, any questionable teeth should be extracted, including wisdom teeth that may present a future problem.

LISTEN TO YOUR DENTIST

Problems with your mouth generally don't get better by themselves. A cavity, crack, or faulty dental work will not repair itself without intervention. We cannot—as yet—grow enamel the same way our nails and hair replenish themselves, nor does gum disease heal spontaneously. It may remain the same for a long period of time, but more likely it will worsen.

One exception is soft tissue trauma. If you burn the roof of your mouth with hot pizza cheese, it may be temporarily painful, but the sore will heal. If you injure your jaw in a fall—and didn't break any bones—it will gradually get better.

In general and by their nature, chronic conditions deteriorate slowly and gradually. But that's not always the case. Disease progression can be variable. I've seen many huge cavities develop from one checkup to the next and well-maintained gum disease worsen in a matter of months. Progression is affected by hygiene, diet, genetics, behavioral habits, and underlying medical conditions. Even stress may play a role, such as causing you to clench your teeth more intensely, deepening a crack.

Not everyone will be like my daughter, whose cavity has remained dormant for years, so the sooner you tend to a problem in your mouth, the simpler, cheaper, and faster it will be. Although conditions can languish for a long time, their course is unpredictable, and what was once a simple fix can turn into an exponentially more complicated and expensive ordeal. For example, a composite resin filling will take one appointment and may run a couple hundred dollars. If that cavity enters the pulp, however, a root canal may be required, followed by a crown. Several long appointments later, you could be facing a $3,000–$4,000 bill.

During a routine visit, your dentist might show you a picture of your chipped filling and recommend its replacement. When you see him six months later, he reminds you about it, then never brings it up again. You might wonder if he made the whole thing up, since he's stopped talking about the chipped filling. Besides, in all that time, it hasn't bothered you. But just because your dentist no longer talks about a problem doesn't mean the issue has resolved. I've been in the exact situation countless times. Not wanting to be "pushy" or sound like a broken record, I have avoided revisiting the problem. I figured the patient would act when he was ready to deal with the issue and I hoped he wouldn't wait until it escalated into a bigger problem.

If you need corroboration, get a second opinion. Bear in mind that some dentists are more conservative in their approach than others. A "let's watch it" cavity for one dentist may be a "must treat" condition for another. It doesn't mean that the more aggressive dentist is treating unnecessarily. A useful strategy is to state up front that you're only seeking a second opinion, and if treatment is recommended, you will have it done elsewhere; this may get you the most objective assessment.

FREQUENTLY ASKED QUESTIONS

Is it true that a tooth with a filling will eventually need a crown?

No, teeth with well-placed and well-maintained fillings—even very large ones—can remain stable for years, if not decades. A crown may be necessary when the filling gets so big that it won't stay in place or be supported by the tooth.

I have a bunch of silver amalgam fillings in my mouth. Should I be concerned about the mercury?

Dental amalgam is made up of silver, tin, copper, and mercury, with the latter being a long-standing subject of controversy. When ingested or inhaled, mercury impairs cognitive function (think of the Mad Hatter in *Alice in Wonderland*). However, research has not shown that mercury exposure from amalgams results in any adverse health effects.[6] Some groups, though, may be more susceptible and should opt for a different filling material. They include:

- Pregnant and nursing women
- Women considering pregnancy
- Children under the age of six
- People with impaired kidney function or neurological illnesses
- People with known metal allergies (this is extremely rare)

How long do fillings last?

Longevity depends on many factors, including the size of the filling, how well it was done, the material, habits such as clenching or grinding, and how cavity prone the patient is. Often a filling needs to be replaced because the patient has developed a cavity adjacent to the existing filling.

Silver amalgam fillings last much longer than tooth-colored composites. (I have some silver fillings in my mouth that are probably forty years old.) Depending on size, composites may be serviceable for five years or so; larger composites will deteriorate faster. A gold filling can last a lifetime.

Why does my tooth hurt after the filling when it didn't bother me before?

With any procedure there can be postoperative discomfort, which disappears after a few days. There can be many reasons for this, but the most common are:

- The bite is high. When you close your teeth together, the new filling is the first point of contact. Go back to your dentist to have the bite adjusted.
- The cavity was really big. Cleaning out decay that is close to the pulp increases the likelihood of irritation and inflammation of the pulp, leading to the possibility of the tooth eventually needing a root canal. In this situation, the best course of action is watchful waiting. Monitor your symptoms. Within six weeks to two months, the tooth should quiet down and the symptoms decrease. If the condition worsens, contact your dentist.
- The filling material irritated the tooth. Bonding agents are used to treat the enamel so that a composite sticks to the tooth and occasionally these chemicals cause discomfort. Symptoms should dissipate within six weeks, so again, it's best to do nothing. Contact your dentist if discomfort persists.

9

OK, I REALLY NEED A CROWN— NOW WHAT?

A crown (or cap) is an artificial tooth that covers over the remaining healthy portion of your own tooth. It is most often needed when extensive cavities leave the underlying tooth too structurally unsound to hold a filling. The crown can preserve the tooth and the integrity of the bite. While crowns should rarely be done for strictly cosmetic reasons, they can be employed to change the shape, size, color, and orientation of a tooth and bring it more into alignment without orthodontically moving the tooth.

As early as 630 BCE, Etruscans living in what is now Italy were using gold in dental appliances to repair and replace teeth. Four thousand years ago, inhabitants of Luzon, an island in the Philippines, modified their teeth by blackening, filing, and using gold. In both cultures, gold was a symbol of status, wealth, and power.

In 1903, Dr. Charles Land introduced the all-porcelain jacket crown, which enveloped the tooth in white. A form of this type of crown is still used today. William Taggart invented a "lost-wax" casting machine in 1907, allowing dentists to create custom-made gold crowns. Even though most crowns aren't made of gold today, they can still cost a significant amount.

CROWN DESIGN

There are basically two options for dental crowns: a full crown and a partial crown. A full crown covers the entire tooth, much like a sock covers a foot. Probably the most common, this kind of crown is quick and easy for an experienced—or even inexperienced—dentist to prepare. Aside from adhering to a few basic principles, the technique doesn't require much planning or thought.

Before installing a full crown, a couple millimeters of the whole tooth—top and sides—must be removed to make room for the crown. From the patient's perspective, this feels like a lot of tooth is drilled away, but the crown materials require a certain thickness to work.

A partial crown is also referred to as an onlay. One of the first tenets dental students learn is the conservation of tooth structure. Enamel is a finite resource, and once it's removed, it is gone forever. The goal of the onlay is to cover only the diseased part of the tooth while leaving as much of the healthy tooth as possible intact. Preparing and installing an onlay requires more thought, precision, and skill than full crowns do. Certainly, it takes more time, and your dentist probably will not get paid more for choosing a conservative onlay over a full crown.

INDICATIONS FOR A CROWN

There are many reasons a crown may be necessary:

- *A large cavity or multiple cavities in the same tooth:* According to standard protocol, when a cavity is treated, a filling is placed. But if the cavity is too large or occurs in multiple areas of the tooth, there may not be sufficient healthy tooth to support and hold such a big filling
- *A defective existing large filling:* Perhaps the most common reason to place a crown is when a tooth with a huge filling or multiple fillings develops a new cavity or when one or more of the fillings is failing.

- *A cracked tooth:* By covering the tooth, the crown is a mechanical solution that braces and holds the pieces together, preventing further breakage.
- *After a root canal:* It is also customary to place a crown on back teeth after a root canal (covered in chapter 10) has been done. A root canal is performed when a tooth's pulp becomes infected. After a root canal, teeth become drier and more prone to breakage, so a crown serves to protect the tooth. In front teeth that are not subjected to heavy biting forces, a filling can often be placed instead of a crown.
- *After an implant:* Crowns are also used as one way to complete an implant (discussed in chapter 11). An implant is an artificial post placed into the jawbone to replace a missing tooth. The implant acts as an artificial root; after it is placed and fuses with the jawbone, a crown must be created to fit on top of it.
- *To change the shape, size, or location of a tooth:* One tooth may be too small in comparison to the rest of the teeth, or perhaps it's misshaped and chipped. Maybe the tooth is sticking out just a tad too much or turned the wrong way, or the color of a previously root-canaled tooth doesn't match the other teeth. A crown can address all these issues.
- *As a foundation for an appliance:* A crown may be needed as a foundation for a partial denture, an appliance that replaces missing teeth. Elements of a partial denture often rest strategically on the surrounding teeth. Or a crown may be required to anchor a bridge, another method of replacing missing teeth. The typical bridge is a unit that consists of a crown on either side connected to one or more artificial teeth.

THE PROCESS

Dentists spend much of their time doing crowns and fillings, so this process is second nature.

The Buildup

After the appropriate anesthetic is administered, the cavity is cleaned out and any defective filling removed. Sometimes this will leave a rather large hole in the tooth, which must be built up prior to continuing.

Some dentists charge separately for this buildup procedure, although it may be argued that it's part of the overall crown process. Sometimes a post (different from an implant) is placed after a root canal, known as a post buildup. With the exception of a post buildup, most insurance plans do not consider the buildup a separate procedure from the crown and will not pay for it. It is important to understand your policy, as you may also be exempt from the additional charge.

The Preparation

In order to make room for the crown, a portion of the tooth—usually around 1–1.5 millimeters of the outside—must be drilled away. Depending on the crown design and material, some crowns require more tooth removal than others.

The Impression

Creating a replica of the prepared tooth is the next step. Most impressions involve the traditional goopy material placed inside your mouth for several minutes, but some dentists use a digital scan in place of the impression material. While this approach is still relatively uncommon, the use of digital scanning is expected to grow. Regardless of the method used, the tooth must be clean and free from any saliva or blood, and the gum cannot cover any of the crown areas.

Most dentists find the impression to be the most challenging—and most critical—part of the whole procedure. Because the crown will be made from the details captured in the impression, it must be accurate. Try to understand if the dentist tells you he has to retake the impression.

The Temporary

Unless your crown will be fabricated while you wait, a temporary crown is used to cover and protect your tooth in the intervening weeks. Because the temporary crown is made from a weaker material than the permanent crown, special care must be taken with it:

- Avoid chewing hard foods.
- Stay away from sticky foods such as gum. Since the temporary needs to be easily removed, a weaker cement is used to hold it in place.
- Do not floss (yes, you heard a dentist say this) in the immediate area; if you must, gently pull the floss out from near the gumline.
- Resist the urge to play with the temporary with your tongue. Even if the temporary is well polished, it will feel rough to our extremely sensitive tongues.
- If the temporary dislodges or falls out, contact your dentist to have it recemented.

The Delivery

Once the crown has been custom made, it is placed and evaluated for proper fit. Often, adjustments to the bite are necessary. The crown is then polished and either cemented or bonded into position.

If you're the type who seeks as much information as possible, there are numerous videos on YouTube that document this procedure. Search under "dental crown" or "dental crown procedure." They are made by dentists, dental laboratories, and even manufacturers of crown materials.

WHAT TO EXPECT

During and after the process, you may experience some common symptoms:

- *Tooth sensitivity:* Your tooth may be temporarily sensitive to temperature or chewing. This sensitivity should spontaneously resolve within days or weeks. If it lingers, this may signal a developing nerve problem.

- *Gum tenderness:* It's not unusual for the gum surrounding the tooth to be tender after the impression. Again, this should spontaneously resolve. On rare occasions, the gum will recede permanently, creating an esthetic dilemma with a front crown. When this happens, the procedure usually has to be redone. If gum recession happens on a back crown that isn't visible, I would advise against repeating the procedure, since any intervention carries a risk of nerve damage to the tooth.

TYPES OF MATERIALS

A discussion of the materials used to make crowns was once simple—and brief. If the tooth was anywhere near the back of your mouth, your dentist would recommend gold. If it was a front tooth, you got either a porcelain fused to metal (PFM) crown or the more aesthetic but fragile porcelain jacket crown.

Now, there are so many materials that even dentists—save for a few dental material nerds—admit to being confused. Just like the latest gadgets, there are unending new variations, each claiming to be superior to its predecessor. However, it's only through time, testing, and observation that new materials can be vetted. Most experienced dentists will wait for this process to occur before embracing every new product.

When my children were young, they delighted in asking their grandfather to open his mouth. Their eyes would widen as they stared at his gold teeth. Sometimes they asked to touch one and inevitably burst into laughter when their finger didn't turn gold. These days everyone wants white. In 2017, approximately 80 percent of all crowns and bridges were some form of metal-free ceramic—in other words, tooth colored or white.[1] When I suggested a solitary gold crown, some patients reacted in horror. Yet there are benefits and disadvantages to all materials.

White (Tooth-Colored) Materials

PFMs　Porcelain by itself breaks easily, but when it is added to the exterior of a metal backing or substructure, the porcelain transforms into a durable and fracture-resistant material. PFM crowns have been used successfully since the 1950s. Until recently, they represented 70 to 80 percent of the crowns made in the United States. Today PFMs make up a scant 17 percent of new crowns.[2]

Despite the material's seventy-year track record and superiority, there is one thing no one likes about PFMs: No matter how well the porcelain covers up the underlying metal, a hint of it is usually visible. When the crown is initially made, this area is tucked under the gum and remains hidden. But even then, depending on the thinness and translucency of the tissue, the metal may cast a grey shadow onto the gum. As the years pass, the gum can recede, revealing the ugly dark line that gives it away—even to the most unobservant person—as a fake tooth.

Lithium Disilicate or E.max　Lithium disilicate, or e.max, has supplanted PFMs in popularity. Since its introduction in 2005, no other material has approached the beauty of e.max. An e.max crown is almost indistinguishable from a natural tooth. Dentists and patients alike love this material.

Your dentist can choose different options with e.max depending on the specific requirements of the crown. More than likely, though, he will delegate the decision to the lab technician. In situations where strength is required, such as a back molar, e.max may not be the best choice, as it may prove too fragile. This material may also be inappropriate for heavy grinders regardless of tooth location.

Zirconia　Fortunately, an even more durable material exists: zirconia. Zirconia—or zirconium oxide—is a relative of cubic zirconia, more commonly known as synthetic diamond. Zirconia is extremely strong, much stronger than porcelain, and has been used in artificial hip joints. In the early 2000s, the first iterations of the material were too opaque to appear natural in the mouth, sticking out like a white blob. Since then, the aesthetics have vastly improved, and zirconia can even be designed as a substructure and combined with an outer layer of porcelain, much like the PFMs.

Initially it was thought that zirconia was much more abrasive than enamel, which would result in premature wearing down of the opposite tooth. However, years of study have proven otherwise.[3] A polished zirconia surface does not wear down enamel, but it is important to have your dentist polish your zirconia crown as necessary. For a heavy grinder, this might be at every cleaning and checkup.

Just as a Honeycrisp is different from a Granny Smith apple, there are many different kinds of zirconia. To name a few, there's 3Y, 4Y, 5Y, and 7Y, each with its own distinct properties. Chances are the average dentist is not familiar with all of zirconia's nuances, but selecting the wrong kind could doom your crown to early failure. The lab technician can be an invaluable resource for your dentist in this matter, which is one more reason for him to maintain a solid working relationship.

Zirconia's strength is also its weakness, though: If the crown ever needs to be replaced, it must first be separated from the tooth, and because zirconia is so tough, it is more difficult and time consuming to drill the old crown off. While more drilling time does not directly cause nerve damage to the tooth, trauma can occur anytime a tooth is worked on and manipulated.

It is clear—to dentists, dental laboratories, dental manufacturers, and the public at large—that tooth-colored crowns are highly desirable and here to stay. While all the materials currently in use have their pros and cons, research is ongoing in the quest to find the perfect, long-lasting dental material that mimics the qualities of enamel and dentin.

Metal Materials

Precious Metals   A precious metal is any rare, naturally occurring element of high economic value. Precious metals used in dentistry are an alloy of gold, platinum, palladium, and silver. Yellow gold contains primarily gold, combined with a mixture of platinum, palladium, silver, copper, and tin to provide the strength lacking in 24-karat gold. White gold has similar ingredients but in different concentrations, resulting in a silver rather than gold color. Both are considered precious metals.

Ironically, we already have a near-perfect material that closely approximates the characteristics of enamel and dentin and has been proven successful over the centuries. That material is yellow gold. One of my greatest joys as a dentist revolves around gold. When I peer into the mouth of a longtime patient and I spot that twenty-five-year-old gold crown, it looks as new and shiny as the day I placed it. Nothing lasts forever, but this comes close. No other restoration holds up as well. Like the feeling a tailor experiences sewing a neckline tag into her creation, that hidden gold crown fills me with a sense of pride and accomplishment. Once, when I presented gold as an option to one patient, almost apologizing that a corner of it might show, she replied, "Well, I'm not a jewelry person, so maybe my gold tooth can be my jewelry."

Aside from the public's desire for a natural, tooth-colored material, the cost of gold has become prohibitive over the years, precluding its extensive use. In 1970, gold was selling for $253 an ounce. By 1980, it had escalated to a whopping $2,000 an ounce. That alone was an impetus for research into more affordable, tooth-colored materials. Although gold prices have fluctuated with economic cycles, as of 2022, gold was selling for around $1,800 an ounce.[4]

Patients familiar with the current price of gold often think their old crowns can be sold for extra cash. While this is true, because the dental gold is a mixture of metals, it must first be separated and purified. The labor to perform this task offsets a sizeable chunk of the expected profit, especially if it's only one crown. Your dentist may keep a jar of discarded gold crowns; when the jar becomes full, the metal can indeed be sold in bulk to metal refiners for extra cash.

Today, yellow gold crowns represent a measly 2.2 percent of all crowns done. Despite this, most dentists—at least ones of a certain age—still maintain that yellow gold is the best material. Many choose it for their own mouths.

The figure for gold crowns increases to over 19 percent if you include PFMs, which utilize a white gold.[5] While it is similar to yellow gold, white gold has a higher platinum and palladium content and is used primarily with PFMs. The porcelain in PFMs must be baked at temperatures that exceed the melting point of yellow gold and thus requires the use of a material that won't melt. White gold is as expensive as yellow gold, if not more so; however, because most of the crown is usually covered by porcelain, less of the metal is needed.

Semiprecious Metals Semiprecious dental metals are alloys containing a smaller percentage of these precious components. Also silver in color, they are used when your dentist wishes to make a less expensive metal crown. As the gold content decreases, the traits that make it dentally attractive—workability, malleability, and biologic compatibility—also decrease.

Nonprecious Metals As the name implies, nonprecious metals contain no gold, platinum, palladium, or silver. Instead, these alloys contain nickel and beryllium, both of which are allergens. Nickel is often found in costume jewelry, but it is also present in many everyday items, such as zippers, coins, and batteries. It is one of the most common causes of contact dermatitis, resulting in itchy, red, and inflamed skin patches. It is also silver in color, so there's no visible way to determine its presence without analysis. But any dentist will tell you that drilling into nonprecious metal is similar to drilling into zirconia: It requires a lot of elbow grease. In spite of any cost savings, nonprecious metals containing allergens have no place inside your mouth.

GOLD VERSUS WHITE

The obvious drawback to gold is just that: It's gold. You may feel differently wearing it around your finger than you do about displaying it in your mouth. There are, however, certain instances in which gold should be considered:

- *Heavy bruxing:* Bruxing is unconscious and repeated grinding of the teeth. Heavy bruxers can wear down teeth, grind holes into fillings and crowns, and fracture ceramic restorations. Gold has a similar hardness to enamel, making it an ideal material.
- *Thin areas:* In the second molar area at the back of the mouth, there is sometimes not enough room for the thickness required to accommodate crowns made of other materials. A too-thin

crown is more likely to fracture or break. Even zirconia, with its minimal thickness requirements, can fracture. Metal almost never fractures and can be cast extremely thin.

- *If the opposite tooth is gold:* If the corresponding tooth above or below has a gold crown, gold is the best choice because crowns made of the same material will wear evenly.

Full disclosure: I admit to being vain. In an area that will not show when I smile, hands down, I would pick gold. Otherwise, I would probably select some form of tooth-colored material. There are pros and cons to each tooth-colored material, and the landscape is continually evolving. Don't micromanage the situation; leave the decision up to your dentist. If it's apparent that your dentist is almost as confused as you are, you may wish to reevaluate the relationship.

The date of a dentist's graduation from dental school may influence his views on many aspects of treatment, including crown materials. Younger dentists may not have received adequate training or exposure to gold, having been educated exclusively on computer-assisted design/computer-assisted manufacturing (CAD/CAM) technology. And after the umpteenth generation of tooth-colored materials, older dentists may have given up on staying current, or they may stubbornly insist that gold is superior. These are obviously generalizations. It is fair to say that dentists—and all doctors—do not recommend what they don't know.

BEHIND THE SCENES

Up until the last couple decades, crowns were made only one way: The dentist sent the impressions to a dental lab technician to fabricate the crown. Most dentists still use outside lab technicians for their dental work. Dentists and lab technicians develop close working relationships, and dentists consult with them on materials and design of the crown, bridge, or denture.

Today, CAD/CAM technology in the form of scanners, milling machines, and 3D printers can also be used to make crowns. Dentists can now offer patients a same-day crown without the annoyance of a temporary or a second appointment. Unless it's a large multidoctor practice or clinic, most dental offices have few employees. One employee cannot be dedicated exclusively to the task of making crowns, so the responsibility falls on the shoulders of the dental assistant, who's already as busy as a short-order breakfast cook. It is important that this person be adequately trained in the CAD/CAM technology and dental anatomy to do a precise and thorough job.

In the movie *Field of Dreams*, the protagonist hears a whisper saying, "If you build it, he will come," urging him to build a baseball diamond in the middle of a cornfield. He's not sure what it all means, but in his heart, he knows it involves a second chance at resolution of past regrets. Your dentist's decision to buy or lease a CAD/CAM machine—costing upward of $50,000—is not as dramatic, but it highlights one thing: The mere presence of the machine may mean that your dentist recommends more crowns. He has a sunk cost, whether it's a monthly lease contract or a lump-sum payment. Or there may be no ulterior profit-driven motive at play; he may simply be excited about this new acquisition. It's up to you to make that assessment.

FREQUENTLY ASKED QUESTIONS

What's the hardest crown to do?

From a purely cosmetic standpoint, the hardest crown to do well is the single upper front tooth. When we look at someone, our eyes are naturally drawn to that spot, and any discrepancy in color or shape between the right and left front teeth (central incisors) will be noticed. Knowing this, some dentists will simply state that you need to crown both front teeth, even though one of them doesn't need a crown. Treasure the dentist who is willing to try to match one front tooth—and understand if it's not perfect.

When getting a crown on a single upper front tooth, what procedure should I consider first?

Before you embark on that treatment, ask yourself if you're satisfied with the color of your teeth. If the answer is no, consider bleaching first. More than once, on the day the patient is to receive a brand-new front crown to replace an unsightly old one, I have heard, "Um, what do you think about the color of my teeth?" The time to ask that question is before the crown has been custom made.

The new crown's color has been carefully matched to your existing teeth. Since it is made of artificial material, not enamel, the crown will not lighten with any bleaching. Bleaching after the new crown is installed will result in a color mismatch. An experienced dentist will prompt this discussion before the procedure begins and allow enough time for the final color to settle down prior to starting the new crown.

What's the most expensive crown to do?

In general, lab bills for crowns are divided into labor and material. There will be a material charge, by weight, for any crown made using a precious metal. As such, even though the labor costs may be lower, gold crowns are the most expensive option for your dentist. One national dental lab charges 3.5 times more for a gold crown than for one made of zirconia. A flat fee is usually charged to make zirconia and e.max crowns, making them much more reasonably priced compared to gold. Add to this the fact that most patients prefer tooth-colored crowns and it becomes an easy sell.

I know most new crowns need to be adjusted, but when is it too much adjustment?

The bite of a new crown frequently requires minor adjustments to make it fit properly and be comfortable in your mouth. In rare instances, patients are so sensitive that they can perceive a .002 millimeter discrepancy in their bite. Once the adjustments are made, the crown is polished and installed. Adjustments taking more than ten or fifteen minutes may distort the shape of the crown, make it more difficult to polish, and weaken the integrity of the material. In a PFM, the porcelain segment can be drilled away so that the metal substructure underneath is showing. Even though the crown is still intact, this may present a cosmetic defect. Every dentist has adjusted a crown so much that a hole is inadvertently created in the crown, automatically rendering it useless. Again, don't micromanage your dentist, but if the adjustment process goes on for too long, understand when your dentist suggests a remake. He's doing so in your best interest.

Why does it matter if my crown is cemented or bonded?

What's the difference between cementing and bonding? With cementing, the restoration is glued onto the tooth. With bonding, both the tooth and the restoration are treated so that a chemical bond and bonding agent keep the restoration attached to the tooth. It produces a much stronger union. In the past, with few exceptions, crowns were cemented and veneers were bonded. Today, materials such as e.max allow for bonding, creating greater retention between the tooth and crown. The problem arises when that e.max crown needs to be replaced: It will take exponentially longer to remove the old crown, with the potential for nerve damage to the underlying tooth.

The decision to bond or cement is, of course, your dentist's responsibility. My rule has always been to bond if it's the only way to keep a crown in place or if the structural integrity of the material requires bonding.

How does insurance factor into all this?

The topic of insurance is covered in depth in chapter 3, but here are a few highlights related specifically to crowns:

- Insurance will typically pay approximately 50 percent for a crown.
- Some policies have a waiting period before paying for any crown.
- If your crown needs to be replaced, most policies will not cover it if the current crown is less than five to eight years old.
- Some policies only pay for metal crowns in the molars. If you pick a white crown, you'll be responsible for any difference in the cost. Ironically, even though that gold crown will cost your dentist much more to make, the insurance amount for gold is

lower than for any of the tooth-colored materials. This is another reason gold is less popular.

- The insurance company will not pay your dentist more for that difficult-to-match front crown.
- There is a distinction between a crown on a natural tooth and one for an implant, which is more expensive.

Why is a crown advertised for so much less elsewhere?

I like to comparison shop as much as the next person, but it's probably not the best way to choose a dentist. Prices differ from one zip code to the next. But if you see a large disparity between fees, you're going to wonder why. Make sure you're comparing apples to apples. The advertised price may be for a nonprecious crown, or perhaps the dentist is sending his work to a lab overseas. Ask questions. What is the experience and skill level of the dentist? What type of lab is being used? How ethical is the dentist?

Why does it seem like my dentist is discouraging me from getting a metal-free crown?

If you're one of the growing number of people who insist on "metal free" in your mouth, ask yourself why. Are you one of the rare individuals who are sensitive to metals? Educate yourself on the properties of the different metals that are commonly used. Understand that *all* materials have advantages and drawbacks.

Any discussion of metals must be specific. Gold and other precious metals are inert and don't interfere with or damage human function or health. Gold leaf (22- to 24-karat gold) is even an ingredient in certain foods. Nonprecious metals such as nickel and beryllium, however, should be avoided.

How long should my crown last?

There are no hard-and-fast statistics, but in my opinion, a crown should last a minimum of five years—and they often last much longer.

There are a number of common factors that contribute to crown failure, some of which have nothing to do with the crown itself.

Any tooth-colored ceramic material can chip or break, and care should be exercised with hard foods like peanut brittle, ice, and the like. However, it's often the initial choice of the material that dooms it. Certain materials are not meant for areas that must sustain the forces involved with heavy chewing. Because of inadequate space, a crown may be too thin and subject to fracture, or the design of a porcelain crown may leave it unsupported and prone to breakage. One frequent scenario is the heavy grinder who insists on having a white material and refuses to wear a night guard. One after another, his crowns break.

When significant breaks occur, a new crown is usually necessary. Occasionally, smaller chips can be repaired or smoothed. Once in a while, a chip can be repaired. With a PFM crown, the metal underneath the porcelain protects the tooth. The crown will need to be replaced only if it becomes a cosmetic problem or the missing area traps a lot of food.

Sometimes a cavity can develop next to the crown, at the vulnerable margin area between the edge of the crown and the tooth, or elsewhere on the tooth. Occasionally this can be repaired, but a new crown may also be indicated. Practice proper dental hygiene to reduce the risk of this happening.

Even with a crown, the tooth or root may fracture. Significant fractures often mean the tooth must be extracted. Or the tooth may become infected, requiring a root canal (discussed in chapter 10) and potentially a new crown. A root canal can often be done through the existing crown by drilling a small access hole.

Sometimes the surrounding area changes, requiring replacement of the crown, for example, if you lose the tooth adjacent to the crown. The decision is then made to fill the missing gap with a bridge, so the crown must be redone as a bridge anchor.

Less severe complications can occur, such as crowns occasionally loosening or coming off entirely. Some dental cements wash out after many years, causing the crown to dislodge. Almost always, a dislodged crown can be cleaned and recemented if you take care of it in a timely manner. A delay of a day or two will not cause problems, but procrastinating longer could mean the difference between simple recementing and a brand-new crown. Whatever you do, stay away from the Krazy Glue and do-it-yourself dentistry.

With certain materials, zirconia in particular, dentists sometimes use the wrong materials to cement a crown, causing it to loosen prematurely. This can also be cleaned and recemented using the proper materials.

If you have a lot of crowns in your mouth, avoid eating sticky foods. Jolly Ranchers, a sticky hard candy, are one of the worst culprits because the candy forces you to open your mouth abruptly.

A crown that is partially loose may be a harbinger of more serious conditions, such as a sizeable cavity growing inside the crown. Another ominous situation is a crown that falls out with the bulk of the tooth inside it. This means that the tooth has broken off at the gumline or a cavity has caused the tooth to deteriorate completely. In either event, the tooth will likely be lost.

Despite all this, with proper planning and care, your crown should last for many years, if not decades.

(10)

WHAT? ROOT CANAL? GUM SURGERY? @#$%?!

Few procedures engender more distaste and fear than root canal and gum surgery. They are viewed as unpleasant, possibly painful, and expensive. Plus, there's nothing tangible—whiter teeth or a new crown—to appreciate afterward. It's the dental equivalent to having plumbing or electrical work done. Hidden behind walls or inside cabinets, they are essential to the operation of the house, but maybe you'd rather have that showcase kitchen instead.

ROOT CANAL

Like hidden passages inside an Egyptian pyramid, an intricate canal system exists inside each tooth, housing the pulp: nerve fibers, blood vessels, and connective tissue. When the pulp becomes diseased, the canals must be cleaned and disinfected, the empty space filled with an inert material. This procedure is called a root canal. But doesn't human tissue need a blood supply? It turns out that a fully mature human tooth can survive indefinitely without a nerve or blood supply. Besides, the tooth receives some nourishment from the surrounding tissues.

Everyone assumes root canals are painful and scary. But with modern anesthetics and techniques, there is no reason for a root canal to be traumatic or uncomfortable. Occasionally an infected tooth will affect the pH of the surrounding tissues by making the environment more acidic, which reduces the effectiveness of the local anesthetic. In such cases, antibiotics are recommended to control the infection before proceeding with the root canal.

Another common misconception is that root canals cause cancer. In the early twentieth century, a dentist named Weston Price conducted a series of flawed tests and concluded that root-canaled teeth harbor harmful toxins that can lead to cancer, arthritis, and other conditions. None of his research results have been proven or duplicated.[1] Yet a century later, in our age of misinformation, this unfortunate myth persists.

Indications

- *A large cavity:* Of the many reasons that warrant a root canal, the most common is a cavity that extends into the pulp of the tooth. Such a large cavity cannot simply be filled. Almost always, the pulp will become inflamed and infected, often leading to intense pain. And there is also the possibility that the infection will affect the rest of the body.
- *A cracked tooth:* Depending on the severity of the crack, a crown may not eliminate all the symptoms. The tooth may still be sensitive to biting or temperature, and sometimes a root canal may help. However, if the crack is too deep, extraction may be the only option.
- *Injury or trauma to the tooth:* Whether from a car accident, a fall, or some other injury, a root canal may be necessary if a chunk of the tooth breaks all the way or close to the pulp. Worse yet, a tooth that is knocked out completely will probably require a root canal if it is to survive. Sometimes the root canal can be performed outside the mouth before reimplanting the tooth. It's easier for the dentist and patient alike!

- A *dead tooth:* Sometimes there may be no symptoms and the patient can't even remember injuring the tooth. The nerve just dies quietly, becoming necrotic and leaving a chronic infection that's diagnosed on a routine X-ray. Or the tooth may darken in color to the point where it obviously contrasts with the other teeth. Left untreated, this infection can grow and cause more harm. After months in quarantine, my ninety-eight-year-old father finally went to the dentist, who discovered a necrotic tooth. Although elderly, he is healthy, and he proceeded with the root canal. It's not uncommon for these chronic infections to flare up when a person becomes sick with some other condition. In his case, being proactive was important.
- *Root resorption:* Another condition that's usually asymptomatic and found on a routine X-ray is resorption. This is a fancy term for a tooth eating away at itself, either internally or from the outside. The condition is not well understood and is thought to possibly stem from past trauma to the tooth. The prognosis for resorption is guarded, but sometimes a root canal is worth a try to save the tooth.

Diagnosis

An unrelenting toothache is often the first indicator that a patient needs a root canal. The patient may complain of spontaneous pain, even when nothing is coming into contact with the tooth. A routine exam and X-ray might reveal the source: a tooth with a large cavity or with an existing defective filling where a cavity has formed around it. Aside from the invasive decay, the tooth is salvageable.

Sometimes there's no apparent reason for the toothache; in fact, the tooth appears totally normal. The dentist must then consider other conditions where the source of the pain originates elsewhere, yet tooth pain is the symptom. The causes may include a different tooth, excessive grinding or clenching, sinus congestion or infection, certain neuralgias, or something unknown. Identifying the culprit can be challenging and involves a fair amount of detective work.

Understand that pain is not constant, even with severe, spontaneous pain. It will exhibit natural highs and lows. When the pain subsides, you might reach the conclusion that the problem has re-solved. But more likely than not, the pain will recur.

Testing

Let's assume the dentist has eliminated other conditions as the causal factor and decides the problem must be coming from a tooth. Now the question is, which one? He reviews the X-rays again, and there's no obvious candidate. There are also multiple teeth with ex-tensive dental work, any of which can be vulnerable due to the previ-ous work. In these teeth, the pulp can become easily inflamed without much warning.

The dentist must test the teeth. As unscientific as this sounds, the diagnosis will be based on the patient's feedback of what hurts. (If you've concluded that modern dentistry should have a more precise method to diagnose pain, I'm in agreement. At the present time, un-fortunately, we don't.)

Since authentic feedback is necessary, it is crucial to avoid taking any pain medication prior to testing, as this will confuse the results. Multiple teeth will be tested on both sides of the mouth to establish a baseline and to rule out referred pain (pain felt in the tooth but origi-nating from another source); for example, a lower tooth may hurt but the culprit is actually an upper one.

The testing involves several modalities:

- *Cold:* Dry ice is usually used to test for a response to cold. In a normal response, you will feel the cold, but the sensation will not hurt or linger. A prolonged sensation can indicate an inflamed pulp. No response whatsoever means the nerve is dead and the tooth needs a root canal.
- *Heat:* A normal response to heat is much like that to cold: You will feel the hot sensation, but it won't hurt or linger. A painful response to heat indicates the nerve is dead. The necrotic pulp creates a gas within the confined canal space and the heat causes the gas to expand, resulting in pain. In this case, a root canal is necessary.

- *Percussion:* A percussion test is usually carried out by a sharp tap with the back of an instrument. Normal responses vary by individual. Some react with surprise, while others barely register any feeling, so it's important to test multiple teeth in addition to the symptomatic one. A sustained painful response indicates an inflamed nerve. It may signal a progression from inflammation to outright infection, necessitating a root canal. Alternatively, as with any bodily inflammation, the tooth could heal by itself and get better.
- *Pressure:* A pressure test involves the gradual exertion of pressure onto the tooth, often delivered by a finger. Like the response to percussion, any positive response can mean inflammation of the tooth.
- *Electrical stimulation:* A device called a pulp tester can be used to send a small electrical current into the tooth. The pulp tester is reliable only for single-rooted front teeth. In teeth with more than one root, parts of the root canal system may be healthy and other areas inflamed or infected, resulting in misleading data. No reaction to the pulp tester indicates the nerve is dead. A weak response may suggest inflammation of the pulp. It's important to test the comparable tooth on the opposite side in the event that you may exhibit an overall weak reaction regardless of the tooth's health. Responses vary by individual, but in general, seniors may have a weaker response. The pulpal system and corresponding nerves tend to shrink as we age. Because of this, any stimulus on the tooth may result in a delayed and/or more muted response. Teeth with crowns or significant dental work may also exhibit a slower and more muted reaction. In cases of trauma, such as recently hitting a tooth on the sidewalk during a fall, responses are unreliable in the first few weeks following the injury. No treatment decision should be made based upon testing results.

Any results of testing must be reproducible and consistent. With ambiguous results, the best action is to do nothing—even if you're in pain—and wait for more definitive symptoms. The dentist must be 100 percent sure of the diagnosis before proceeding with a root canal. There have been cases in patients with trigeminal neuralgia where sequential root canals have been done in error when both the patient and dentist assumed the source of the pain was from a tooth.

Sometimes the dentist can determine that you need a root canal based solely on X-rays or the condition of the tooth, without performing any tests. The challenge will be to convince you because you have no symptoms. Besides my father's example, I've come across huge cavities that should be painful but aren't; however, when they think back, almost all patients will recall past episodes of pain from the decayed tooth. As the cavity progresses, the tooth can become quietly necrotic. With a dead nerve, there won't be any sensation, but the infection is present and can cause serious harm—in rare instances, it can even lead to death.

You may be asking yourself, "If there's an infection in my tooth, why can't I simply take antibiotics to cure it?" For antibiotics to work, they must travel through the bloodstream to reach the source of the infection. Because they are surrounded by bone, teeth are in a particularly hard-to-reach spot. Antibiotics may help if the infection is acute and causes swelling into the gums. They may make you feel better temporarily. But medication alone will not eliminate the infection at the base of the root next to the bone.

The Process

To begin a root canal, the dentist first numbs the tooth. After the tooth is numb, a five- or six-inch square of latex called a rubber or dental dam is placed over the tooth to isolate it from the rest of your mouth and keep it dry. The dentist drills a small opening in the tooth, locates the canals, and calculates their precise length. She then cleans and shapes the canals, after which they are filled with an inert material called gutta percha. Finally, she places a temporary filling to protect the opening. A root canal can be done through an existing crown, assuming the crown fits properly and is otherwise serviceable. A small hole is drilled into the crown and later patched with a filling once the root canal is done. This demands a higher skill level, so it may be advisable to see a specialist.

Root canals used to drag on for at least two appointments, but now most are completed in one. In part the philosophy has evolved and, with some exceptions, dentists no longer see the need for the tooth to heal in between appointments. Getting a root canal these days is remarkably quick.

The process has also become more efficient as a result of innovative new equipment. High-quality root canals can be done without such equipment, but they make the task easier. One is the apex locator. Each canal must be cleaned to its terminal point, but not beyond it. Dentists have traditionally used X-rays and clinical experience to figure out where this spot is, but the apex locator calculates the exact stopping point automatically. Another useful piece of equipment is the microscope. While most dentists work with 2.5- to 5-times magnification attached to their glasses, the microscope used for root canals can magnify up to 25 times. Commercially introduced about thirty years ago, these microscopes are used by the majority of root canal specialists (endodontists) today. They also use motorized rotary instruments to clean and shape the canals. In the past, only tiny doll-like hand instruments called files were used. Hand files are still popular, but the rotary ones make the process less tedious and time consuming.

In rare instances, the human body performs its own root canal. Ordinarily the canal system is evident on an X-ray as an empty dark space. After, say, a sports injury or car accident, the body can heal itself. When this phenomenon occurs, the canal system disappears and turns whitish on the X-ray, filled with the cementum that comprises the root portion of the tooth. The canal space becomes indistinguishable from the surrounding root. When questioned, the patient may recall some traumatic incident from the distant past.

What to Expect after the Root Canal

You may feel fine after your root canal, or you may experience some common symptoms.

- *Pain:* You thought the root canal was the solution to your toothache, but you're still having pain (although it's reduced). Or your tooth may have been asymptomatic before, and now it hurts. It's normal to experience pain or discomfort for twenty-four to forty-eight hours after the procedure. Beyond that initial period, the pain should dissipate. If it doesn't, contact your dentist.

- *Inability to chew:* The tooth can be sensitive to chewing for several weeks—or even months, in rare cases—after the root canal. It can also be tender if you press on the tooth with your finger. Contact your dentist if this sensitivity persists.
- *Swelling:* The area around the tooth may become swollen, possibly indicating an infection. Contact your dentist if this happens.

Next Steps

- Baby the temporary. There's probably a temporary filling in the tooth. Use extra caution not to dislodge it. Chew on the other side of your mouth.
- Eat soft foods. If you're experiencing pain or tenderness, stick to a soft diet for the next few days.
- Additional procedures may be necessary. The tooth becomes drier and more brittle following a root canal. Shortly after its completion, a crown is typically recommended to protect the tooth from breakage. Get the crown done as soon as possible to prevent further bacterial contamination. As discussed in chapter 9, before the crown can be installed, what's left of the remaining tooth must be reconstructed or built up. A post may be used to anchor the buildup if there is insufficient healthy tooth. If a specialist has done your root canal, she may also handle the buildup, or your dentist may do it. Sometimes, a permanent filling will suffice in lieu of a crown. This is common practice in a front tooth where the bulk of it is intact and healthy.

Root canals are remarkably successful, with rates approaching 90 percent.[2] If a root canal fails, it will not be right away; often it's years later. At that point, a retreatment—redoing the original root canal—may be considered, although the chances of success are lower. Retreatments generally require greater skill and experience as the old gutta percha filling must be removed and the canals cleaned properly.

Saving the Tooth versus Extraction

Faced with a tooth needing a root canal, you may be thinking: Why don't I just pull the tooth and save myself thousands of dollars? Consider this: It will be equally expensive, maybe more so, to replace the missing gap with an artificial tooth.

What about just leaving the space? While it's true that your chewing and speech won't be impacted by one missing tooth, the space can potentially cause a series of adverse bite changes. The tooth behind the gap will lean forward like the Tower of Pisa, resulting in periodontal problems. The tooth in front of the gap may drift backward, leaving an annoying space between it and its neighbor. Food may get stuck there after every meal, again creating a gum problem. The tooth above the empty space may move down; in the worst case, it won't stop until it reaches the bottom gum. (The reverse, teeth moving up, generally doesn't happen with the same frequency.)

If multiple back teeth are missing, the entire bite can collapse, putting unreasonable strain on the front teeth and the temporomandibular joints. The front teeth may loosen and flare. Without the back teeth touching, the TMJ are forced into an unnatural position, potentially causing joint damage and muscle fatigue. Often, when patients finally decide to fix their teeth, so much shifting has occurred that it's now an engineering nightmare, with exponentially higher costs. And sometimes perfectly healthy teeth have to be sacrificed because they've moved too far and have become obstacles.

In the last hundred years, views on extraction have changed. In 1916, psychiatrist Dr. Henry Cotton, the superintendent of Trenton State Hospital in New Jersey, was convinced that dental infections were the cause of mental illness. He proceeded to conduct wholesale extractions of teeth. Unfortunately, his patients' mental health didn't improve.

One of my first patients in dental school was "Patricia," a woman in her seventies who had all her teeth pulled out at the age of twenty-one. This unthinkable yet commonplace practice was a "gift" to her so that she wouldn't incur a lifetime of dental expenses. What Patricia couldn't anticipate were the decades of discomfort she would suffer from eating with dentures as her gums shrank. By the time she turned seventy, there was nothing for her dentures to grab onto for stability, and the lower in particular caused problems as it moved around in her mouth.

Dentists now try to save teeth whenever possible. Tooth loss among older adults has decreased significantly. With the exception of "hopeless" teeth that require major reconstruction offering unpredictable outcomes, dentists believe in preserving natural teeth. Still, about one in six adults over the age of sixty-five has lost all their teeth.[3] Edentulism—having no teeth—is unfortunately tied to poverty, lack of education, and smoking. The advent and popularity of implants (discussed in chapter 11) has shifted thinking about tooth preservation slightly; in certain instances, an implant may be viewed as having a greater likelihood of long-term success.

SO WHAT SHOULD YOU DO?

The question of which option to choose is a complicated one, and the short answer is: It depends. Each situation is unique—and often there's no single right answer. Begin by asking the following questions:

- What is required to restore the tooth? Besides the root canal and crown, are there additional procedures necessary, such as gum surgery (in this case, a procedure called crown lengthening) or a post buildup? Consider the overall costs and timeline.
- How healthy is the tooth? The tooth may be compromised by existing gum problems, or perhaps more than half of the top portion of the tooth is gone or severely decayed. The less structurally sound the tooth is, the greater the risk of a restorative failure.
- If the tooth is extracted, what procedures will be required afterward? This could be something simple and affordable like adding a fake tooth to an existing partial denture. At the other end of the spectrum, reconstruction might mean an implant and an implant crown with its associated parts. Again, review the overall costs and timeline.

Consider contributing factors. What is the condition of the rest of your mouth? So far, we've been addressing individual teeth, but sometimes a decision is made considering all your teeth as one unit. Maybe multiple teeth require root canals and crowns, or perhaps there is gum disease throughout. What is your dentist's assessment of your mouth in totality? How does this tooth relate to the overall plan?

Perhaps there are medical conditions that would favor one option over another. For example, a patient with dry mouth who is more prone to decay may prefer a cavity-immune artificial implant and crown, whereas someone who has undergone radiation treatment will do everything possible to retain the tooth to prevent the risk of osteonecrosis.

Your dental hygiene should also be considered. Are you able to keep your teeth clean? This is a prerequisite to any major dental work. Otherwise, it may be a waste of time and money.

Regardless of whether the tooth is extracted or restored, all major dental procedures are expensive. If cost is a limiting factor, discuss this with your dentist. There are always creative ways to spread out the procedures while still maintaining quality and a high degree of success.

Don't assume that you're "too old" to invest in your mouth. You may need a root canal on a pivotal anchor tooth for your partial denture, an appliance that replaces some missing teeth. If that crucial tooth were to be extracted, your partial denture would become wobblier, making eating much more difficult. On the flip side, even if a tooth is structurally weak, a root canal and crown may be the best option for a still-growing young person. Placing an implant before a patient is physically mature results in problems later.

Whatever you do, to prevent serious cascading events, don't just pull the tooth—and nothing more.

PERIODONTAL (GUM) DISEASE

Each tooth in your mouth sits inside your jawbone, anchored by tiny ligaments that connect the root(s) to the bone. The gum drapes over the bone, much like a glove covers your hand. If the bone shrinks, less of the tooth will be supported and the tooth will loosen. The gum may shrink along with the bone, resulting in gum recession, but more often it remains, like loose skin on an aging torso. This excess gum creates crevices—or pockets—where bacteria can proliferate. Plaque, the sticky whitish/yellowish substance that forms around your teeth, contains mostly bacteria and can be brushed off. But once plaque hardens, it turns into tartar (calculus), and must be scraped off. The tartar attaches itself to root surfaces deep inside the pockets, further inhibiting your ability to clean your teeth effectively.

This creates a vicious cycle: The body mounts an inflammatory response to rid itself of the microorganisms trapped within the tartar and plaque, and as a result of this response, the supporting jawbone may be gradually destroyed as your body's immune response attacks the bacteria. Then, as the bone shrinks, the pocket becomes deeper and the tooth progressively loosens. Other times an outright acute infection occurs, also damaging the bone and leaving a wiggly tooth.

We call this gum disease. Dentists refer to it as periodontal disease or periodontitis. But it's really an infection affecting the gum and, more critically, the bone and tooth inside the gum. Its precursor is gingivitis, a term you may have heard in toothpaste advertisements. While the name sounds scary, gingivitis is actually the earliest, mildest, and *reversible* stage of gum disease. Technically, we all have some gingivitis. It stems from not brushing and flossing adequately and shows up as red, puffy, and bleeding gums. Gingivitis can occur on isolated teeth or throughout the mouth, and with good oral hygiene habits, it can be reversed and the gums will return to normal.

In the United States, 47 percent of adults over age thirty have some form of gum disease; it is second only to cavities as a common oral health problem. The occurrence of periodontal disease increases with age; 70 percent of people over age sixty-five show signs of the condition.[4] In 2018, according to a *Journal of Periodontology* analysis, the indirect cost of periodontal disease was estimated at $154 billion.[5] That includes productivity losses from someone calling in sick due to gum problems and from distracted workers making mistakes because their mouth hurts.

As with other diseases, there are several risk factors:

- *Age:* Gum disease is a slow, chronic condition. In its early stages, there are often no symptoms, and consequently, it's easy to ignore. This may be one reason we see more gum disease in older populations.

- *Smoking:* Tobacco use represents one of the principal risk factors in gum disease, as well as other conditions such as oral cancer. Smoking is also cited as a major reason for implant failure.
- *Stress:* Stress is linked to many health conditions, but the mechanism remains poorly understood. I have seen many patients whose gum disease has been well controlled for years but worsens drastically in a matter of months. When questioned, most of these patients describe a recent stressful episode in their lives. One specific gum disease caused by stress is called acute necrotizing ulcerative gingivitis (ANUG), or trench mouth. The name originated from the many soldiers in World War I who developed this condition in the trenches. ANUG is characterized by sudden onset of painful gum sores and distinctive breath odor. It is caused by a combination of poor oral hygiene, poor diet, and lack of sleep, but the primary factor is stress. ANUG is also seen in college students during exam weeks. With proper hygiene and rest, it usually resolves on its own.
- *Overall health:* Systemic conditions such as diabetes, cardiovascular disease, cancer, and dementia show a link to gum disease, but again, the connection is not completely understood.
- *Genetics:* Although rare, children can exhibit aggressive forms of gum disease caused by genetic factors. Despite treatment and good oral hygiene, many teeth become loose, and the long-term outlook for retaining teeth is poor.
- *Medications:* Certain medications can affect gum health. Any medication that induces dry mouth—and there are many—increases risk of gum disease. Other medications cause growth (hypertrophy) of the gums.
- *Grinding or clenching:* Oral habits such as grinding or clenching that place undue pressure and force on the teeth increase the risk of gum disease, often resulting in loose teeth.
- *Socioeconomic factors:* Poverty, malnutrition, and obesity form a complex web of interrelated risk and challenges for gum and overall oral health.

The Mouth-Body Connection

We're learning more and more that the health of the mouth and the body are interrelated. Some systemic diseases are linked to periodontal disease. People with diabetes, for example, are more likely to suffer from gum disease, and periodontal disease makes it more difficult for diabetics to control their blood sugar. The relationship between the two appears to be circular.

With cardiovascular (heart) disease, the relationship is less clear, although there is a documented link between heart disease, stroke, and gum disease. Adults with gum disease may be significantly more likely to have high blood pressure. With respiratory diseases, bacteria found in gum disease can be aspirated and lodge in the lungs, causing pneumonia. One recent study revealed that people with severe gum disease were three times more likely to experience severe COVID-19 complications such as ICU admission and assisted ventilation.[6] In osteoporosis, which primarily affects postmenopausal women, the density of the jawbones is reduced, resulting in a less solid foundation for the teeth.

Periodontal disease may also be influenced by gender. Women experience hormonal swings throughout life, especially during puberty and menopause. These swings can cause gums to become easily irritated, swollen, and bleed more. The same gum changes can occur during menstruation. Over the years, countless women have told me that a tooth that bothers them occasionally will flare up right before or during their periods. The same is true during pregnancy: An old wives' tale says that with each pregnancy, a woman loses a tooth. While that's not the case, there are definite hormonal changes and a marked increase in blood volume, so thorough oral hygiene is critical to counteract swollen or bleeding gums. It's a good idea for pregnant women to get their teeth cleaned once, if not twice, during pregnancy. Pregnant women with active periodontal disease are more likely to have premature births, so it's critical to treat and gain control over the gum disease.[7] As for menopause and beyond, women may experience dry mouth, burning sensations, and altered taste to salty, peppery, or sour. Postmenopausal women may also be taking more medications, many of which contribute to dry mouth.

Men, for reasons unknown, have more gum disease than women: 56.4 percent versus 38.4 percent. Men with gum disease are also 49 percent more likely to develop kidney cancer, 54 percent more susceptible to pancreatic cancer, and 30 percent more likely to suffer from blood cancers. Men with periodontal disease are also at greater risk of developing impotence.[8] Chronic inflammation appears to be the underlying factor.

Recent research points to inflammation as the common denominator among some systemic diseases.[9] Simply put, inflammation is your body's immune response to an irritant. Whether it's a bug bite or a bacterial infection, the body enlists an army of white blood cells to fight it off. Sometimes the immune system goes into overdrive and continues to fight after the irritant has already been subdued. Alternatively, the immune system may inadvertently destroy the body's own good cells, as is seen in the bone destruction of gum disease, joint damage in rheumatoid arthritis, and skin lesions in psoriasis.

Before Symptoms Appear

In its early stages, gum disease will show no symptoms. That's why it's critical to get routine periodontal exams (discussed in chapter 4), which include checking each tooth for mobility; evaluating the gums for bleeding, recession, and texture; a bite evaluation; and detailed pocket charting. Be forewarned—many patients find pocket charting uncomfortable. In this exercise, an instrument is placed between the tooth and gum; you will hear your dentist or hygienist call out a series of numbers such as "323, 222, . . ." and so on. Any number greater than 5 millimeters merits a discussion. It means you have a pocket—a space that's too deep for you to adequately clean, where microorganisms can live and proliferate. (And you thought deep pockets were a good thing . . .) It's been shown that a toothbrush can clean, at most, 3 millimeters below the gumline[10]—about an eighth of an inch. So it's virtually impossible for you to clean the base of a 7-millimeter pocket. Consequently, bacteria thrive in the pocket and the surrounding bone may be destroyed, making the pocket even deeper. Eventually, the pocket is so deep that the tooth feels loose, pus and swelling may occur, and pain ensues. By that time, extraction is the only option.

Make sure your dentist or hygienist is not only measuring the pockets but also discussing the findings and, most importantly, treating and managing any periodontal disease. There have been cases where a new dentist takes over a retiring dentist's practice only to discover that no plan other than "watchful waiting" has been established for the patients with a mouthful of pockets and gum disease. It's no wonder that lawsuits alleging a dentist's failure to diagnose periodontal disease often result in some of the highest settlements.

Signs and Symptoms

Periodontal disease is a slow, chronic condition, and it may take months or even years for symptoms to appear. The symptoms can be isolated to one or a few teeth or affect the entire dentition. If you experience any of these signs and symptoms, see your dentist:

- Bleeding during brushing or eating
- Red, swollen, or tender gums
- New gaps in your teeth or a change in the way your teeth fit together; both indicate tooth movement
- Flaring of your front teeth
- Loose teeth
- Persistent bad breath; the odor from active periodontal disease is unique and should be easily recognizable by your dentist
- Pus seeping from your gums

Treatment and Management

There are a number of ways to treat periodontal disease, but they all share the same goals: to control or eliminate the underlying cause—the bacterial population—and to create an environment that allows the patient to keep the area clean. Due to its chronic nature, in addition to treatment, periodontal disease must be managed throughout a patient's lifetime.

Treatment is divided between nonsurgical and surgical approaches. A conservative approach is typically best, and most treatment will begin with nonsurgical methods. Additionally, before gum surgery is considered, it's important that you can demonstrate proficiency in cleaning your mouth. Otherwise, the expense and effort of the surgery are wasted and your gum disease will recur.

Nonsurgical Treatment   Scaling and root planing—or deep cleaning—is the first step in treating gum disease. It is tedious and time consuming, and usually half or a quarter (quadrant) of the mouth is treated at one appointment. Scaling and root planing is done by either the dentist or the dental hygienist using hand instruments, ultrasonic cleaners, or lasers. Occasionally, microscopes are even used to better visualize the tartar below the gum. Almost always, local anesthetic is administered. In scaling and root planing, tartar and plaque are scraped off the tooth, leaving a smooth surface that is resistant to bacteria. The subgingival tartar—that is, tartar found below the gum—can be extremely stubborn and challenging to remove. It is an expensive process, particularly if you have the mindset that you're "just getting a cleaning." Most insurance policies will cover the bulk of the costs, but increasingly, insurers want to see evidence of gum disease through X-rays and documentation.

If done properly, two things will happen after scaling and root planing: The bacterial count will be reduced and controlled, and the pockets will shrink in depth so it's easier for you to clean. From your perspective, it will seem like the longest teeth cleaning you've ever had. Your mouth will be sore afterward, and your teeth may be sensitive to temperature for weeks. As the gums heal, you may notice new gaps between the teeth and gums—areas that now trap food. They may be unsightly, appearing as tiny "black holes" in your mouth. You may even feel like the treatment is worse than the disease. After all, you didn't have any of these symptoms prior to the deep cleaning. But rest assured that the sensitivity will diminish and disappear. The spaces will remain, but it's a small price to pay for good gum health. If they continue to bother you, once your periodontal condition stabilizes and you can demonstrate good oral hygiene, you can discuss cosmetic options with your dentist.

All scaling and root-planing procedures should include a follow-up appointment where the pockets are measured and evaluated for improvement. Further, you must be instructed on how to perform good oral hygiene so that you have the tools to prevent gum disease from recurring. An appraisal of how well you're cleaning should be part of the follow-up.

Gum Surgery   Sometimes the pocket reduction will be less than expected, and depending on the severity of the gum disease, often there has already been bone loss. Remember that the gum drapes over the bone. If there are small defects and crevices in the bone architecture, the gum cannot follow the contours of those defects. A vacuum will be left—a perfect place for bacteria to set up housekeeping. In those instances, gum surgery may be the next step. During gum surgery, part of the gum is removed to make the pocket shallower. You must be prepared for how this will look—where gum used to cover the teeth, there may now be many gaps. Keep in mind that this will help you retain your natural teeth.

Currently we can grow bone, and even teeth, in a laboratory setting. The teeth, however, come out as undifferentiated blobs. In the future we may be able to grow bone in the mouth. For now, we have bone grafts at our disposal, and this is routinely employed during gum surgery. Bone grafts come from various sources: your own body (autograft), cadaver tissue (allograft), animal bone (xenograft), or synthetic materials (alloplast). With the aid of graft materials, membranes, and growth-stimulating proteins, regenerating bone in isolated defects has been successful. In this way, bone lost in gum disease can be replaced.

Although traditional surgery involves the use of a scalpel, lasers are now playing a larger role in dentistry. Despite any skepticism on the part of dentists, lasers have been used effectively in the treatment of gum disease. Their results are comparable to traditional surgical methods. But like all techniques, the dentist's skill, knowledge, and experience in choosing a laser over more conventional methods are critical.

Adjunctive Therapy

There are other treatments that may help in the battle against periodontal disease. Adjunctive in nature, these measures play a supporting role, but will not eliminate the condition. A word of caution: There are harmful and beneficial bacteria in the mouth microbiome. Any non-specific antibiotic or bactericidal rinse, such as chlorhexidine or bleach, will also reduce the beneficial bacteria. Consult with your dentist and physician first.

- *Localized antibiotic delivery:* An antibiotic can be placed directly inside a pocket to manage the bacterial content. This is usually done in conjunction with scaling and root planing.
- *Systemic antibiotics:* Aggressive cases of gum disease may benefit from a round of orally adminstered systemic antibiotics. Testing can be done to identify the offending groups of bacteria in order to select the appropriate antibiotic. This is usually administered before starting comprehensive scaling and root planing. The therapeutic effects of antibiotics are short-lived, and the micro-organisms will multiply again if the source of infection is not removed. To help control chronic cases, sometimes low-dose antibiotics are periodically prescribed. The risk of antibiotic overuse and bacterial resistance are important considerations.
- *An old-fashioned home remedy:* In lieu of antibiotics, an inexpensive way to control bacteria is rinsing for thirty seconds twice a week with diluted .25 percent sodium hypochlorite[11]—household bleach. Sodium hypochlorite has been used as an antibacterial agent since the nineteenth century. Standard household bleach is 6 percent concentration. Double-check the math—please—but that works out to two teaspoons in one cup (eight ounces) of water.[12] Be sure to use unscented bleach and try delivering this solution through a water flosser.
- *Rinsing with chlorhexidine:* Chlorhexidine is a prescription antibacterial rinse, used primarily as a short-term measure for patients after an invasive dental procedure such as gum surgery. Longer-term use results in stained teeth and altered taste sensation.
- *Fluoride trays:* Gum surgery often leaves portions of the roots exposed. Since periodontal disease happens more often in older people—who may have reduced saliva flow from medications—the roots become vulnerable to decay. Fluoride gel administered via trays offers some level of protection.
- *Occlusal adjustment:* As part of the periodontal exam, the bite should be checked. An ideal bite is one where the teeth touch evenly upon closing. When you move your lower jaw right or left, as happens in chewing, there should be no teeth that bang into one another, with the exception of the canines. Any deviation from this ideal can negatively affect the periodontal health of the

teeth. An occlusal adjustment—or bite adjustment—brings your bite to ideal. It usually involves minor grinding of certain teeth. Although enamel is finite, the removal of specific areas of enamel is warranted in this situation.

- *More frequent cleanings:* Without exception, any patient who has undergone recent scaling and root planing or gum surgery should have their teeth cleaned every three to four months. Even though most insurance plans cover only two cleanings annually, some will extend this to three with proper documentation from your dentist.

- *Oral hygiene instruction:* It takes time to teach someone a new skill and involves watching and critiquing as necessary. Let's face it: Your dentist doesn't get paid to do this, and most offices do a cursory job. Consider offering to pay for this service. Your ability to maintain your periodontal health on a daily basis is critical. Gum disease is not like a cavity that once filled can be forgotten. It is a chronic condition and bacteria live inside your mouth. Without adequate hygiene, the pocket depths will recur.

- *Diabetes control:* Gum disease and diabetes are closely linked. If one is uncontrolled, the other will suffer as well.

- *Smoking cessation:* Smoking is a major risk factor on multiple health fronts. Aside from the physical addiction, there's the overwhelming psychological aspect. Ask for help if you need it. There are many smoking cessation programs.

Unrelated Gum Procedures

There are other gum procedures that have nothing to do with periodontal disease but can be useful in correcting other problems.

Gum Grafting   Think of this as the opposite of a pocket. Rather than reducing the depth of the pocket, gum is added to cover areas where there's been recession. Grafting is done for numerous reasons:

- *Cosmetics:* Receding gums lengthen the visible portion of the tooth and expose the root, which is usually a darker color. This can make us look and feel old. Covering the receded area with a gum graft results in a more youthful appearance.

- *Tooth sensitivity:* The root surfaces can be extremely sensitive to hot, cold, and even spicy foods. Gum grafting is one technique to eliminate this sensitivity.
- *Improving the quality of the gum:* Sometimes the tissue around the root is thin and fragile, or it may not adhere well to the root surface. By grafting material, the area is reinforced and further gum recession is prevented.

Just like bone grafts, gum grafts can come from various sources. One common area is from the palate. Gum is harvested from the roof of your mouth and transplanted. Expect some discomfort in the donor area afterward. Another area is from the neighboring tooth. Like sharing a blanket, gum can be split and grafted from the adjacent tooth. There must be tissue thick enough to share, though. Finally, an allograft from another person can be obtained through a tissue bank.

The most successful grafting is done in the early stages of gum recession. If the grafting is attempted in the later stages, the graft will not last. Avoid such a disappointment by addressing the problem early.

Crown Lengthening   As the name implies, crown lengthening is a procedure that makes the visible part of the tooth longer. Generally both a section of the gum and the supporting bone must be removed. Crown lengthening is never done as an isolated procedure. The most common reason for this procedure involves a single tooth where a crown is planned. There may be a cavity below the gumline that needs to be exposed. For a successful crown, all the decay must be accessible and visible for the buildup and crown preparation. Sometimes a cavity is not the impetus for crown lengthening; rather, the tooth is simply too short and there's not enough tooth above the gum to hold a crown. After the surgery, the gum is allowed to heal for several weeks, after which the crown is started.

Crown lengthening may also be indicated before cosmetic reconstruction. Some people naturally have small teeth that almost look like baby teeth. Others present with a "gummy" smile. Crown lengthening will make all the teeth longer and more full-bodied and grown-up in appearance. Because this involves multiple teeth, possibly a whole row, there is usually some discomfort afterward.

Frenectomy   There are a half dozen muscle attachments in the mouth. If one is too close to the surrounding teeth, it can damage the gum and eventually the tooth. A frenectomy entails moving the muscle attachment away from the tooth.

Sometimes frenectomies are done prior to orthodontic treatment to relocate a muscle attachment so teeth can be moved. Frenectomies are also performed in infants and children to eliminate tongue-tie. (This will be discussed in chapter 12.)

A FINAL WORD

Root canal and gum surgery are really about managing infection, inflammation, and our continuing struggle with harmful microorganisms. These treatments contribute not only to our oral health, but our overall health, and their importance cannot be overstated.

11

I HAVE MISSING TEETH—ARE IMPLANTS THE WAY TO GO?

Imagine you had a root canal done years ago, and now it's painful and infected. In a scene that plays out daily in dental offices across the country, your dentist informs you that the tooth cannot be saved. He may automatically say, "You need an implant," but there are several options to replace the missing tooth or teeth: the implant and implant crown, a bridge, or a partial denture. The decision should be made on a case-by-case basis.

OPTIONS TO REPLACE MISSING TEETH

The Implant

The implant is a treatment option where the replacement feels and acts like a real tooth and is essentially an artificial root to replace a missing tooth and is embedded into the jawbone. Surrounded by bone and covered over with gum, it is not visible. Connected to the implant is either a crown, a bridge, or a denture. An implant is often—but not always—the best choice. An implant should be considered under the following circumstances:

- The teeth on either side of the diseased tooth are healthy with no major dental work.
- The implant must be surrounded by strong, healthy bone, so adequate bone is a prerequisite. If bone grafting is required to add additional bone, the procedure must demonstrate a high likelihood of success.
- There is adequate space—width and length—for the implant and crown. Sometimes this can be corrected orthodontically, but the additional treatment time and cost may be prohibitive.
- The patient's mouth and jaws are fully grown and physically mature. Note that boys develop later than girls and may not be fully grown until age twenty-five.
- There are no systemic conditions, such as serious autoimmune illness, that would greatly reduce the chances of implant success.

The beauty of an implant is that after the initial adjustment, you'll probably forget you have one in your mouth because it will feel like a natural tooth. The implant is easy to clean, and you can brush and floss it like the rest of your teeth. A negative to this expensive procedure is that the entire process—from the extraction of an infected tooth to the final crown placement—is lengthy. For those with dental insurance, there may be a silver lining: Because the time may span across two calendar years, portions of the treatment can be billed in different years to take full advantage of your benefits. A larger negative is that implant failures are costly to correct.

The Bridge

A bridge—two crowns on either side with an artificial tooth (or teeth) in the middle, all in a single piece—should be considered under the following conditions:

- There is existing dental work on the anchor teeth at either end, either crowns or large fillings. These teeth should be otherwise healthy, with no periodontal problems or vulnerable root canals.

Since drilling is done on the anchor teeth, using perfectly healthy teeth is not recommended.

- The patient's medical history or young age prevents her from getting an implant. (Notice I didn't mention old age, which by itself should not be a metric.)
- There are anatomical deficiencies that make implant placement difficult, such as inadequate space, insufficient bone, or gum defects. The correction will be significant and likely impractical.
- The patient cannot tolerate the idea of something artificial imbedded into her body.

Doing a bridge is a much quicker process than an implant. After a four- to six-week healing period from the extraction, the bridge can be started and completed in as little as one day to two weeks. The process is equivalent to doing a crown (discussed in chapter 9). In contrast to the implant, the entire process takes two months rather than six to nine months. A bridge is also generally cheaper than an implant and implant crown. In situations with a pronounced gum defect, a bridge provides more versatility in terms of masking the defect.

One drawback is that because the bridge consists of multiple teeth in one unit, it is more difficult to clean. Special floss threaders (discussed in chapter 6) are used to clean between the teeth in the bridge.

The Partial Denture

What we call a partial denture may really be one of two different things. It may be a permanent appliance, like a full denture but replacing fewer teeth. A stayplate—affectionately known as a "flipper"—can be thought of as a temporary partial denture. It performs the same function but is made of less durable components. In either case, the partial denture is fully removable.

A partial denture is the ideal choice if you already have a partial denture and are accustomed to wearing one. An additional tooth can be added quickly and inexpensively. The process for making a new partial or full denture involves a series of approximately six short appointments, typically without the need for anesthetic.

A flipper is indicated in the following situations:

- The patient is too young for an implant and wants to wait for one.
- Due to financial reasons, the patient cannot commit to either the implant or the bridge currently. The flipper is then used as a temporary treatment.

A removable appliance is easy to clean: You simply take it out and clean it, then brush and floss your teeth as you normally would. A partial denture is also by far the most affordable option. However, partial dentures and stayplates do not feel like natural teeth, and there may be psychological implications associated with wearing false teeth. They tend to make people feel old. To varying degrees, the appliances move around during chewing and food can lodge underneath. Occasionally, taste is compromised. And because they are removable, appliances can be misplaced or lost.

IMPLANTS—IN DETAIL

Every year, more than eight hundred thousand individual implants are placed in the United States. In spite of the significant costs— upward of $4,000 per implant, not including the final crown—the popularity of implants continues to rise. This growth is attributable to an increasing older population, more widespread implant knowledge and training among dentists, and greater awareness of implants within the general population. In the period between 2006 and 2016, implant placement multiplied fourfold. During the same time span, the placement of new lower partial dentures decreased by over 40 percent. It's no surprise that people have traded in their partial dentures for implant restorations.

The earliest evidence of dental implants was discovered in Mayan civilizations from around 600 CE, where they used pieces of shells to replace lower teeth. In the 1930s, two brothers, Drs. Alvin and Moses Strock, placed the first endosseous implant—an implant within the bone—using a biocompatible chrome cobalt alloy that had been used successfully in hip implants. In 1978, Dr. Per-Ingvar Brånemark, a physician and researcher considered the father of the modern dental implant, developed a titanium endosseous dental implant. In experiments studying blood flow, he placed titanium in rabbit femurs and accidentally discovered that the material bonded to the bone in a matter of months, so much so that the titanium couldn't be removed. Since then, titanium has remained the material of choice for dental implants.

A naturally occurring chemical element, titanium can be found in abundance in China and Australia. Silver in color, titanium has high strength, low density, and resistance to corrosion. Because it doesn't corrode, titanium doesn't leach into the body, nor do bodily fluids weaken its integrity, making it a truly biocompatible material. Titanium's unique ability to physically bond to bone gives it another advantage. No adhesive is required to keep the implant attached. Its high strength—comparable to steel—is perfectly suited to the forces found in chewing.

For patients who have metal sensitivity or allergy, zirconia—the same material often used in crowns—is a relatively new alternative. Although it was approved by the Food and Drug Administration (FDA) in 2011, its use has been limited in the United States. Zirconia is biocompatible, aesthetic, and integrates well within the jawbone, but it is weaker than titanium, posing a higher risk of implant fracture. There are also fewer options for designing and attaching the final crown, bridge, or denture. More research needs to be conducted on the long-term viability and success of zirconia implants.

There are several indications for implants. They include:

- *To replace missing teeth:* This is the most common reason for implants, which can be used to replace a single missing tooth, multiple teeth, or an edentulous mouth.
- *To replace damaged or missing body parts:* Implants can be employed to attach prostheses. For example, with cleft palate, a retainer-like prosthesis re-creates the normal anatomy of the roof of the mouth, and implants can assist in holding the prosthesis in place. Brånemark placed an implant behind the ear of a hearing-impaired thalidomide adolescent so that a novel hearing aid could be attached.

- *As anchorage in orthodontic treatment:* A temporary, smaller sized implant can be placed in the gum to assist with the movement of teeth during treatment with braces. The implant supplies an additional counterweight to move teeth through dense bone.

Choosing an Implant

The fact is that patients have very little input into the choice of implant; your dentist will be the one making the choice. When there's a surgeon involved, the dentist may defer to her in making this decision. Still, it's imperative that you have a general idea of the implants available so you understand what's going in your mouth.

All implant manufacturers sell some variation of the titanium implant. There are more than a hundred implant companies, but only a half dozen or so major ones. Think of them as the Mercedes of the dental implant world—and these companies produce high quality, higher priced implants. As of 2021, the top implant companies in the United States are:

- Straumann—A Swiss company, Straumann is involved in many areas of dentistry in addition to its implants.
- Envista—This is the parent company of numerous dental entities, most notably Nobel Biocare and Implant Direct. Nobel Biocare is the company that launched the original Brånemark implant, whereas Implant Direct is a maker of low-cost implants.
- Dentsply Sirona—This is a multifaceted dental company. Besides Astra implants, they make a variety of dental equipment and consumable products. Interestingly, they've recently acquired MIS Implants, an Israeli maker of "value" low-cost implants.
- BioHorizons—This company is known for their innovative implant products and extensive research.
- ZimVie (formerly Zimmer Biomet)—ZimVie primarily deals with dental and spine related products.

These are all multinational companies with a worldwide audience. They deal with products across the entire dental industry. As for implants, there's an ongoing subtle shift toward recognition of a more value-based, lower-priced production. (Note that some of the companies listed above also have lower-priced lines that are marketed separately.) Perhaps this will signal a decline in the high cost of implant restoration. Be skeptical, though, of an implant that is advertised at too low a price; it's probably too good to be true. But what is so special about the implants from these manufacturers that would warrant quadruple the price tag when the material is virtually the same? After all, the implant is buried inside the bone and under the gum. There are several reasons why it pays to select one of these implants:

- *Manufacturer longevity:* Despite mergers and changes in ownership via acquisitions, these companies have been in business for a long time, which means they are more likely to remain in business. One implant company, Zimmer Biomet, was founded in 1927. Longevity equates to a greater likelihood there will be spare parts and tools available should you need it. The company will also have long-term data on the performance of their products.
- *Research and development:* Major implant companies have a larger percentage of the implant market. With their substantial revenue and size, they can maintain research and development divisions. As a result, these companies have been responsible for marked improvements in implant design and have originated novel ways to treat the titanium for greater success. Using their products provides patients with these advantages.
- *Support:* Many of these companies have dedicated field representatives that can assist your dentist. When I did my first implant crown, the rep sat in the room and walked me through the whole procedure. A live person is also available by telephone for questions. If your dentist is unfamiliar with the specifics of an implant, there is a source for support. These companies often sponsor courses to train dentists on their products.
- *Familiarity:* If a product or company is well-known, more dentists and lab technicians will be knowledgeable in the product's use. There is also a greater probability that most dentists or lab

technicians will stock the tools necessary for the implant, making it easier to repair or replace a broken implant later.

- *Product warranties:* Some companies provide lifetime guarantees on their products, provided no aftermarket parts have been used, the procedure was done properly, and the patient treated the implant reasonably.

The Process

Ask anyone who's ever had an implant and they will likely say, "I had no idea it would take so long." From the time the tooth is extracted until the crown or denture is installed, the implant process can take nine months, sometimes longer if extensive bone grafting is required.

Planning and Preliminary Work The first step is planning. With replacement of a single tooth, an examination, X-rays or scans, and a review of options may be all that's needed. A complex case involving multiple implants will require more thought: Where are the ideal locations for implant placement? Will more than one doctor be involved? If the implant is to anchor a denture, will it be permanently attached onto the implants, or will the patient be able to remove the denture nightly to clean underneath?

Sometimes there may be preliminary procedures that need to be done before the implants can be placed. These can include bone or gum grafting, a surgical procedure to trigger the body's own ability to create more bone, or an orthodontic procedure to maximize bone level. This may involve seeing multiple specialists.

The Extraction You may be sweating already, picturing a cartoon of a sadistic dentist, feet braced against the dental chair, yanking the forceps back and forth in a frenzied attempt to pull the tooth. Take a deep breath. It's not like that anymore. When an implant will be placed, teeth are extracted atraumatically—gently, with as little disturbance to the surrounding gum and bone as possible, using special instruments that have been designed for this purpose.

Implant Placement After the extraction, one of two approaches will be taken: Either the implant will be inserted right away (immediate placement), or the socket will be allowed to heal for several months and the implant will be installed after healing is complete (delayed placement). In the 1980s, when implants first gained traction in the United States, delayed placement was standard protocol. Now both methods are accepted and the decision about timing should be made on a case-by-case basis.

Immediate Implant Placement Immediate placement will shorten the time frame by three months, but it can be employed only under certain conditions. First, there must be sufficient bone to lock in the implant. Because the shape of the implant differs from that of the root, granules of bone filler are packed into the remaining voids. In addition to quantity, the quality of the bone must be considered. Compared to the upper jaw, the bone in a lower jaw is denser, making it a better candidate for immediate implant placement.

A significant infection will also preclude immediate placement, but a small chronic infection, such as from an old root canal, may not present an issue.

For the dentist, placing an implant right away may be more technically challenging. Further, some dentists prefer taking the more conservative approach of letting the socket area heal.

Patient compliance is also important. Putting any pressure on the implant during the months it takes for the implant to fuse with the bone can significantly reduce the chances of a successful outcome. You cannot chew near the implant site. It's one thing to hear this guidance, but adhering to it—meal after meal—is another story. Infrequently, the temporary is removed after three to four months only to discover that the implant is loose. At that point, you're essentially starting over. The loose implant must be taken out and, after a three-month healing period, another implant is placed.

Delayed Implant Placement With delayed placement, sometimes the dentist will cover the entire implant with gum, uncovering it after the three- to six-month osseointegration period, when the implant bonds to the bone. Other times the top of the implant will be exposed and protected with a metal cap—a healing abutment—much like the top in a jar of jam.

During the Osseointegration Period After the implant is placed, regardless of approach, the area is left alone. In the lower jaw, this is a period of three to four months, while in the more porous upper jaw, it can stretch from four to six months. What happens in those intervening months? Is it similar to a crown procedure, where you get a temporary? Not necessarily. Mostly it depends on the location of the space.

In the posterior (or back) of the mouth, almost always, you'll live with a gap. It may drive your tongue crazy until you get used to it, and when you finally get the implant crown, there will be another adjustment period for your tongue. During this time, there may be the possibility of a top tooth supraerupting, or growing down into the empty space below it. This will make placing the eventual implant crown more challenging. The reverse—a lower tooth drifting up—rarely occurs. Although it isn't standard procedure, you may want to consider a retainer to avoid this.

In the anterior (or front) of the mouth, a temporary is almost always placed. It may be a temporary tooth attached directly to the healing implant. Patients love this option because it feels the most natural. That said, manage your aesthetic expectations, as the temporary tooth will be smaller than the final crown. It will definitely not touch any of your other teeth when you bite together, but even so, extreme caution must be exercised to not chew in this area. In the critical cosmetic zone of the upper front teeth, the temporary serves to shape the surrounding gum so that it's symmetrical, full, and ideal.

After several months, this temporary tooth will show its age. Nevertheless, if the implant is on the upper front teeth, consider saving the temporary in the event that the permanent implant crown needs to be repaired or remade at some point. While a new temporary can also be fabricated, having the old one will save some inconvenience and money.

Alternatively, you may receive a flipper. This is a retainer with one or more false teeth attached to the acrylic. Most people hate this appliance and use it only for appearance. In the privacy of their homes, they take the flipper out prior to eating to avoid the annoyance of getting food trapped underneath. The flipper may alter speech and interfere with the ability to taste. Despite all its drawbacks, if you have a flipper, consider saving it as well for future contingencies.

What about the premolar teeth at the sides of the mouth that may show when you talk or smile? Since these are technically back teeth, dentists are reluctant—with good reason—to attach a temporary tooth to a healing implant. Chewing forces, particularly lateral (side-to-side) ones, can adversely affect the integration of the implant to bone. So in these premolar teeth areas where the gap may show, a flipper may be your only choice. You may feel that the flipper is mandatory. In my experience, almost every patient who has invested in a flipper for this area eventually stops wearing it. They either train themselves not to smile as broadly or they get to the point where they don't care if the gap shows, but either way, the flipper ends up in a drawer.

People with no teeth obviously need a temporary denture. These patients may have an existing denture or partial denture that can be modified for temporary use. On the other hand, a patient who is scheduled for a mouthful of extractions and multiple implant placements will need a set of interim dentures fabricated beforehand.

The Permanent Implant Restoration

After months of waiting and postoperative appointments, the surgeon has finally pronounced your implant ready to restore. Your general dentist may not be the one who placed the implant, but most people return to their dentist for the final restoration, whether it is a crown, a bridge, or a denture.

The Implant Crown or Bridge   An implant crown is an artificial tooth attached to the implant. An implant bridge is typically one or more artificial teeth anchored by an implant crown on either side. An implant bridge should not be anchored by a natural tooth on one end and an implant on the other. In specific situations, the bridge may be cantilevered, meaning it is anchored to an implant only on one side. Regardless of whether the final restoration is a crown or bridge, the process is identical. What's more, the materials used—metals, porcelain, e.max, and zirconia—are the same as those used in the fabrication of a crown (described in chapter 9). The lab procedures, while not identical, are comparable. In the posterior area, the restoration may be a bit smaller than your natural teeth. This minimizes undue forces, reduces porcelain fracture, and may increase the long-term success of the implant.

Cemented versus Screw Retained   Your implant crown or bridge will be one of two designs: cemented or screw retained. While being educated about the options is important so that you understand what you're getting in your mouth, ultimately, the design of the restoration will be up to your dentist. She will decide whether your implant crown or bridge will be cemented or screw retained. Technical nuances beyond the scope of this discussion and your dentist's individual preference will guide the decision.

The cemented implant crown or bridge looks just like a crown that would fit over your natural teeth. Adhesive cement is used to keep it in place. Because the implant ends at the gumline, an additional component called the abutment is screwed into the implant and used to hold the crown in place, acting much the same as a natural prepared tooth under the crown. Created from metal or zirconia, the abutment can be either custom made or stock purchased from the manufacturer. Although they are more expensive, custom abutments, created by lab technicians, are preferred to produce a more ideal crown or bridge.

Cemented restorations can be done in any situation. For your dentist, the process is just like restoring a natural tooth. Cemented restorations are also cheaper to make than screw-retained ones. Once cemented, these restorations are not easily retrievable. If something breaks, repairing it often entails remaking the entire crown or bridge, and sometimes the abutments as well. Your dentist must also be extra careful not to leave any excess cement under the gum, which can lead to peri-implantitis, an inflammation of the gums that may compromise the long-term success of the implant.

With the screw-retained crown or bridge, the restoration is in one piece rather than two. The abutment is combined with the crown or bridge into a singular unit, and the entire thing is screwed into the implant through a small hole (or holes in the case of a bridge) in the middle of the restoration. Afterward, a filling is placed to cover up the hole. Depending on the position of the implant relative to the tooth, not every restoration can be done this way. In cases where the screw hole would exit through the outer surface of the crown or bridge, creating an unsightly obstacle, a cemented restoration is the only option.

The biggest advantage to screw-retained restoration is retrievability. By removing the filling and the screw, the restoration can be removed for repair or in the event it needs to be remade. Also since no cement is needed to hold it in place, potential problems with cement hidden under the gum are eliminated. However, the screw-retained crown or bridge is more expensive to make. It is also more tedious for the dentist to adjust and polish the restoration. The sheer bulk of material makes it more prone to porcelain fracture, so the design of the restoration must be thoughtfully planned out by the lab technician. Screw loosening is also an annoying problem. Finally, after investing so much time and money, some patients don't like the hole in the middle of their new implant crown or bridge, even when it's in an area that's not visible. Many patients want their restoration to look just like a brand-new tooth.

The Implant Denture Without a doubt, implants have dramatically improved the quality of life of denture wearers. Rather than enduring a diet of soft foods, they can look forward to eating foods they enjoyed in the past. There are two treatment options for implant dentures: the removable or the screw retained.

Removable implant dentures look remarkably similar to conventional dentures. On the underside, though, there are indentations that correspond to the location of the implants. The denture fits onto these implants to provide additional stability, allowing it to stay in place better. The connection between the denture and implants isn't fixed; in other words, there's wiggle room. Just like taking off your shoes and socks at night, the denture can be removed to "air out" the underlying gums. The implants can then be brushed and cleaned before bedtime.

Screw-retained dentures mimic real teeth, for the first time allowing denture wearers the capability to re-create what they've lost. These dentures are attached solidly onto the implants with screws and can be removed only by the dentist. In the upper arch, the palate is eliminated in favor of a horseshoe-shaped appliance, allowing patients to taste their food without a barrier of pink acrylic. The process involves approximately ten implants and corresponding parts. It's a complex engineering project carried out by a team that includes the dentist or prosthodontist (a specialty discussed in chapter 13), the surgeon, and the lab technician. Screw-retained dentures can cost as much as a luxury automobile, but for many, it's well worth the price to regain the feel of natural teeth.

Factors Contributing to Implant Success

Implants enjoy a high degree of success. Most studies place the success rate between 90 and 95 percent.[2] Well-considered decisions and proper execution of the numerous factors involved account for this success.

Overall Health   The first consideration begins with an assessment of your overall health. Are you immunocompromised? Do you suffer from advanced heart disease, diabetes, or another major systemic illness? If so, you're not an ideal candidate for an implant. Do you smoke? Initially, dentists were discouraged from placing implants in smokers, but now, you simply have to acknowledge the risk that your implant has a greater chance of failing.

Oral Habits   Do you grind your teeth intensely over sustained periods of time (heavy bruxing)? That will also compromise the likelihood of success. If you brux at night, are you willing to wear a night guard to protect the implant and corresponding restoration?

Quantity and Quality of the Surrounding Bone   It would be great if implants could be placed randomly in areas of plentiful bone, after which your dentist could create beautiful, functional teeth. Unfortunately, that's not the case. Following the rules of biomechanics, implants should be placed so they are only subjected to vertical chewing forces rather than lateral ones. In situations with insufficient or inadequate bone, placing the implant in a less than ideal position compromises its success. So does choosing an implant that is shorter or narrower than desired, as the implant may be less stable or fracture.

Proper Technique   This almost goes without saying that proper surgical and clinical technique is paramount, including adherence to a sterile environment. With implant placement, for instance, the bone cannot be overheated and must be irrigated with saline. Proper selection and fabrication of the restoration is equally important. Because of these factors, having the work done by skilled surgeons and dentists increases the chances of success.

Proper Bite Adjustment   The major difference between an implant tooth and a real tooth is that the implant has no shock absorber. In a real tooth, the periodontal ligament (PDL) separates the root from the surrounding bone. Despite its name, the PDL is actually a collection of tiny fibers that connect the root to the bone and provide the "give" to accommodate our masticatory forces. The implant, by contrast, is fused to the bone—and immovable. The difference is much like that between the cushion in a pair of running shoes and the stiff sole of dress shoes.

Because there is no PDL around the implant, the single most important thing is the bite. Your dentist must adjust the bite meticulously. Some dentists prefer to err on the side of caution, intentionally making the implant crown shorter so it doesn't touch the opposing teeth. However, for the time and money invested, I believe the restoration should be as precise as possible—and that includes the bite.

Potential Complications

Peri-implantitis Think of peri-implantitis as gum disease of your implant rather than your natural tooth. It is the most common complication, affecting approximately 5 to 8 percent of implants over their lifespan.[3]

With peri-implantitis, the gum around the implant becomes inflamed. At this point, the condition is referred to as mucositis—and, like gingivitis, it is reversible. As the condition progresses, the supporting bone around the implant slowly disappears. Depending on the severity, peri-implantitis doesn't automatically doom the implant. Often it can be treated and managed, just like periodontal disease. However, if it is left untreated, the implant may eventually loosen and become infected, requiring removal.

The same risk factors that predispose individuals to gum disease apply to peri-implantitis. These include poor oral hygiene, smoking, and diabetes. Excess hidden cement under the gum is another cause; it acts as an irritant, attracting unwanted plaque and producing an inflammatory reaction.

Fracture Although infrequent, any of the components—the implant, the abutment, or the screw—can fracture or break. For screw fractures, provided the screw can be retrieved without damaging the other parts, it is an easy fix to replace the screw. Abutment fractures necessitate replacing the abutment, screw, and crown or bridge. A postmortem should be conducted to identify the cause so that this rare mishap doesn't occur again. Regrettably, implant fractures mean starting from scratch and replacing everything. Most fractured implants are solidly integrated into the surrounding bone, presenting a technical challenge for removal.

In the past, a technique called trephination—where a section of bone is cored out around the implant—was exclusively used to remove a broken implant. Because healthy bone is intimately connected to the now-unusable implant, trephination removes a healthy portion of the bone along with the implant. In recent years, reverse torque drivers have been developed that can unscrew a fractured implant with minimal destruction of the surrounding bone. This method offers a clear advantage over trephination.

Rejection by the Body   In rare instances, there's no identifiable reason for implant failure. One day the patient simply notices the implant crown is loose. The gum appears healthy, and there's no mechanical break or any problem with the residual cement or the crown itself. In this poorly understood process, the implant may have been gradually rejected by the patient's own body.

When this happens a first time, because the causes cannot be accurately identified, it's reasonable for patients to repeat the implant process. With multiple failures, patients must consider alternative options, such as a bridge or partial denture.

Restoration Failure   A much more common occurrence is the breakdown of the final restoration. In particular, fractures in porcelain and other tooth-colored material are often seen with crowns and bridges. Sometimes, an entire section of the restoration will be sheared off.

It can be a big deal to replace the implant crown or bridge. For cemented crowns, sometimes the abutment must also be replaced. For both screw-retained and cemented restorations, a new screw is required. (A new screw directly from the manufacturer was priced at $50 pre-COVID; aftermarket knockoffs are less expensive but may void any warranties.) There are specific tools that your dentist may need to purchase or borrow if the implant manufacturer is not one she routinely works with. Impression and laboratory parts must also be obtained. The costs add up quickly.

Occasionally, repairing the crown or bridge may be an option. As with a chipped crown on a natural tooth, creative ways exist to repair a small to moderate porcelain fracture. If the restoration is in the posterior and doesn't interfere with eating or speaking, smoothing and polishing the broken area may be all that's needed.

Porcelain fractures generally stem from two causes: Either the restoration was designed incorrectly such that the porcelain isn't properly supported, or the bite is off. In comparison to a natural tooth with a PDL, the bite on an implant crown is much less forgiving. Periodically—maybe once a year—the bite should be evaluated for any changes and the crown adjusted and polished accordingly. The changes may be so minor that you're unaware of them. Don't balk if your dentist charges you for this service, as his attention to it now could save you from a much greater expense down the road.

Implant Failure

Implants generally fail at two times: within the first six months or after years of service.

Early failure is often discovered when your dentist begins the final restoration. You may experience pain as the impression parts are placed into the implant, indicating that the implant has not fully integrated or bonded to the bone. It may be loose, but regardless, the implant must be removed. Then, after three months of healing, the process can be repeated with a new implant. While it's impossible to pinpoint a culprit, premature loading of forces on the implant is often implicated. Chances are you were inadvertently chewing in that area. A variation on this early failure is the implant that falls out spontaneously within days of its placement. In this case, there just wasn't enough bone to hold the implant.

Late failures, on the other hand, happen years after the implant treatment, during which time the implant and restoration have been functioning problem free. In late failures, almost always everything— the implant, the implant restoration, bone grafting, gum grafting—has to be redone. Nobody likes to see a late failure, as it is emotionally, financially, and physically stressful. But it happens.

When a failure occurs, who is responsible? With multiple components and parties involved, it is often impossible—and impractical—to assign blame. For example, if a spicule of cement is discovered under the gum, can we be absolutely certain that is what caused the implant to loosen? Even if the excess cement was the culprit, your dentist may have done everything humanly possible to remove the cement. Or perhaps the position of the implant precluded the possibility of a screw-retained crown, in which case, maybe the surgeon is at fault. Or insufficient bone—not surgical skill—may be the reason the implant was placed the way it was. The situation can become muddled quickly.

Most dentists are reasonable in early failure cases. After such an investment, your implant shouldn't fail before the crown is even started. With delayed failure, it can be argued that you've enjoyed many good years of service. Your dentist may decide that paying for a new implant and crown should be your responsibility.

Essential Details

You've invested in a high-quality implant from a reputable manufacturer. After months of waiting, you're finally getting the implant crown. It will feel fabulous to have a tooth again. There's one last task: You need to obtain certain essential information from your dentist, who may not be proactive and volunteer this material.

Record the Specifications   Ask for a record of the manufacturer, type of implant, and size. Without this information, it will be very difficult to figure out any of the particulars of your implant, especially if it came from a little-known company. You may believe that since your dentist has this information, there's no reason for you to have it. But patients move and change dentists, professionals retire, and records get destroyed. This information is crucial if you had implants placed overseas during a dental tourism trip.

Get a Photo   If you have a cemented crown, insist on a photograph of the abutment showing the location of the screw. In the event the crown chips, this picture will make it easier to identify the screw's position so the crown and abutment can be removed for repair. To take this one step further, I even had the lab mark the exact spot on the crown. Trying to locate the screw blindly results in indiscriminate drilling that can compromise the integrity of the abutment or crown.

Keep the Temporary Even if it's seen better days, your temporary crown or flipper will come in handy in the event you need to have the restoration remade.

For the Super Planners . . .

Those who thrive on being prepared may want to pay for the necessary parts required to make a new crown in the event that years from now, these parts may be discontinued. Of course, this depends on the confidence you and your dentist have in the implant company and its commitment to support older products. Discuss this further with your dentist or surgeon.

Reasons to Delay Implant Therapy

If you're considering orthodontic treatment in the near future, do that first before embarking on an implant. The PDL makes it possible for teeth to move, and its absence in implants prevents them from moving. Unless the implant is placed in the ideal after-braces spot, it will create spacing problems.

Few situations are black and white, and perhaps there's a possibility your tooth can be saved. Often it's a toss-up between doing a root canal and crown versus extraction and an implant. Provided finances are manageable, try to maintain your natural tooth first. It's remarkable how long a loose or weak tooth can last. Even if it means redoing it later with an eventual implant, you'll have bought yourself some time during which technology may have improved.

If you were purchasing a car forty years ago, a gas- or diesel-powered vehicle was your only option. Now we can choose from hybrid, electric, and hydrogen-powered cars. As it does with automobiles, implant technology continues to evolve—and it may even change faster because it's a newer product. While it's perfectly acceptable for someone in their twenties to get an implant, keep in mind that in fifty years, the implant landscape may be completely different. If you have a baby tooth with no permanent successor, for example, consider holding on to that tooth as long as possible. (Some of my patients had baby teeth well into their sixties.)

Finally, remember this: Implants are a replacement for natural teeth, but no implant can take the place of a natural tooth.

FREQUENTLY ASKED QUESTIONS

I have periodontal disease and some of my teeth feel loose. Should my implant feel loose as well?

Because the implant is solidly bonded to the bone, it should never feel loose. Contact your dentist right away. There may be several possibilities:

- The implant itself is loose.
- The crown is loose.
- The screw has untightened and needs to be replaced or retightened.
- One of the components—the implant or abutment—has fractured.

Depending on the findings, the remedy may range from minor to complicated.

I got an implant a few years ago. Recently I have been getting food stuck there every time I eat. Should I be concerned?

In a process known as mesial migration, posterior teeth tend to move toward the center of the mouth over time. But without the PDL, the implant does not move. Mesial migration can result in an irritating space between the mesial aspect (the side of the implant closest to the center of the mouth) and the natural tooth directly in front of it. While the implant crown cannot get a cavity, the natural tooth can. Both the natural tooth and the implant "tooth" can potentially suffer from gum disease and peri-implantitis, respectively. Even with a screw-retained crown, there are limitations to correcting this problem. While the crown can be removed and adjusted, additions of porcelain are usually not effective after a crown has been in acidic oral fluids for years. At this point, diligent oral hygiene may be the only solution.

Why does my implant suddenly seem shorter?

Teeth move passively over time. Besides mesial migration, there is another natural tendency for teeth to elongate and continue erupting. If this happens in the upper front area, you may observe the implant crown appearing shorter than the neighboring teeth. The issue isn't the implant crown; it's the other teeth that have moved. One potential solution to this is recontouring and shortening the other teeth to match the implant tooth. Alternatively, the implant crown can be redone. (This is where you'll be glad you saved the temporary.) Of course, a third option is to leave it as is.

You shouldn't be able to see your implant, should you?

As discussed earlier in this chapter, implants can suffer from mucositis and peri-implantitis, resulting in gum and bone recession. Sometimes this process can be treated and return to a stable plateau. Unfortunately, if gum recession has already occurred, the top greyish threads of the implant will be visible. If the area doesn't show unless you lift your lip, the best course of action is to do nothing. In a highly visible, critical area, the options for remediation may be frustrating, limited, and expensive. Gum and bone grafting can be attempted, possibly entailing removal of the implant. Or the implant may have to be abandoned for another treatment strategy.

My pacemaker and even my washer and dryer have serial numbers. Why doesn't my implant have one?

You're right: Pacemakers, orthopedic prostheses, and most major appliances have serial numbers. Why should dental implants be any different? A serial number would go a long way in determining the exact nature of the implant. If this information were kept in a national database, it could even assist with forensic identification.

(12)

KIDS AND SENIORS—TWO ENDS OF A SPECTRUM

SENIORS

In 2018, more than one in every seven Americans was an older adult. Every day in the United States, ten thousand people turn sixty-five, accounting for 16.5 percent of the population. That number is expected to increase as the population of baby boomers ages. But seniors are by no means a demographically homogeneous group. Many between the ages of sixty-five and seventy-four are still working, actively involved in society, and capable of managing their dental needs. Contrast this to the eighty-five-and-older population, the group which requires the most care: Their numbers are projected to double from 2018 to 2040.[1]

About one in six older adults has lost all their teeth (edentulous). Despite the growing number of seniors, the rate of edentulism is actually decreasing in the United States. Since the 1999–2004 period, edentulism has dropped by 10 percent.[2] Still, that's a lot of people with no teeth. Within this group, there's huge variation. You're much more likely to be edentulous if you're a smoker, live in poverty, or have less than a high school education.

If you're over age sixty-five, chances are you may be missing an isolated tooth here and there. But with some knowledge and good care, you'll likely keep most of your teeth through your lifetime.

Changes as We Age

Aside from greying hair, wrinkles, and loss of muscle mass, there are changes inside our mouths as we age. Other changes directly affect our dental and overall health. Still other developments are cosmetic, but they influence our general outlook and how we view ourselves as we get older.

- *Bone loss:* Even in a relatively healthy mouth free of acute gum disease, there may be gradual bone loss with age. This translates to less of the tooth held securely in bone, potentially contributing to tooth mobility. In addition, women—and some men—experience a decrease in bone density as they age; in women this is especially true after menopause.
- *Gum recession:* Since the contours of the gums follow the shape of the underlying bone, gum recession becomes more prevalent with age. This may leave empty spaces in between the teeth, areas where food particles can remain after a meal. Anyone over a certain age will attest to this annoying development. Referred to as black triangles in the visible front teeth, these spaces can also be mistaken for lingering food remnants. Gum recession may also expose the roots of teeth, which are more prone to cavities since root surfaces are not protected by enamel. The darker color of the roots may also present a cosmetic issue.
- *Structural wear of the teeth:* With decades of use, teeth get worn down, becoming flatter and shorter. The enamel may get thinner, and the underlying dentin may even be exposed. Teeth may chip with greater frequency. They may break more easily, sometimes completely shearing off at the gumline, particularly if the majority of the tooth consists of dental work.
- *Yellowing or darkening of the teeth:* Because of their porosity, teeth absorb everything we eat and drink. Smoking, coffee or red wine, and highly colored foods contribute to this.

- *Increased crowding of teeth:* Over time, teeth have a tendency to move toward the center of the mouth. As such, the lower front teeth become more crowded, trapping more food and making oral hygiene more difficult. This potentially leads to more bone loss and gum recession.
- *Relaxation of facial muscles:* When a twenty-one-year-old smiles, the upper teeth show and the edges follow the contour of the lower lip. As skin and muscle tone loosens over time, the lower teeth are more likely to be displayed. Depending on the wear of the teeth, sometimes hardly any teeth show during speech or in a smile. Although primarily a cosmetic issue, this may make an older person appear guarded or even angry.
- *Side effects from medication use:* People under the age of thirty-five fill an average of three prescriptions annually. For the population over age sixty-five, this can increase to more than twenty prescriptions.[3] Many medications have significant side effects, such as dry mouth, which impact oral health.
- *Decline in manual dexterity:* Just when oral hygiene becomes more critical, difficulties with manual dexterity can make it more difficult to execute it properly.
- *Cognitive decline:* Under the best of circumstances, it can be challenging to interact with a healthcare provider in the brief time allotted for an appointment. With any cognitive decline, information can be misinterpreted or confused. It may be difficult to make treatment decisions or understand the dentist's instructions regarding post-treatment care.

Recommendations for Home Care

Individuals age at different rates and have different needs. Some of these recommendations may not be applicable now but could be relevant as a senior progresses from sixty-five to eighty-five:

- Avoid extremely hard foods. Think twice before biting into that piece of peanut brittle or chomping on an ice cube. (This actually applies to all age groups.) Why risk having a chunk of your tooth break off?

- Use fluoride products. The combination of dry mouth and gum recession puts the roots at risk for hard-to-treat cavities to develop. Fluoride can help protect against tooth decay.
- Dislodge trapped food particles. Consider rinsing after every meal to remove food particles. A water flosser is extremely useful in helping to remove food debris between the teeth.
- Consider investing in an electric toothbrush, especially if manual dexterity is compromised. Research shows electric toothbrushes clean more effectively than manual brushes.
- Use Biotene for dry mouth. No product can fully eliminate dry mouth, but the Biotene products are useful for this purpose. It's also important to drink plenty of water.
- Use Stain Away Plus for cleaning dentures. Again, no product will remove all the stubborn stains that form on a denture or retainer. Stain Away Plus does a good job. If the appliance has tartar formation, take it to your dentist to be professionally cleaned.
- Consider a walking stick. An increasing risk as seniors age, falls can result in broken teeth and other bodily injuries. A walking stick is a simple way to prevent unnecessary trauma and expense.

Recommendations for Professional Care

Just as overall health issues increase with age, dental problems also generally become more common, and it can be daunting to deal with necessary treatment. Perhaps you tire easily; if so, ask for shorter appointments earlier in the day. If you are like many seniors living on a budget, speak to your dentist about alternative treatment options. Formulate a realistic plan together to address your dental needs. Maybe you have mobility issues. There are mobile dentists who make house calls; they come equipped with handheld X-ray units and portable drills.

General recommendations for dental care in older adults include:

- Get regular exams and cleanings. During routine exams, your dentist will be able to identify concerns as they develop. Once a problem escalates, it will prove more difficult and costly to manage.

- Consider a fluoride treatment. After your cleaning, ask about a fluoride varnish treatment. In the United States, fluoride treatments for adults are generally not covered by insurance, but they should be. Fluoride is an inexpensive, effective means to prevent cavities. For vulnerable patient groups, fluoride can be a powerful therapeutic ally.
- Bring a friend. It's always helpful to have another set of eyes and ears at a medical appointment. As your patient advocate, the other person can take notes, ask questions, and clarify the subject as needed.
- Take notes. To fully understand and retain what is being said during the appointment, take notes or record the conversation. Also, have the office staff give you the treatment recommendations in writing. In my experience, some patients, elderly or otherwise, will bring a notepad and write down information. A few of these may be in the early stages of dementia. A skilled dentist should recognize this and, in addition to clear explanations, provide pamphlets and drawings to enhance understanding.
- Don't forget to get hearing and vision exams. While this doesn't relate strictly to dental health, an inability to see well impacts all areas of your life, including your ability to perform oral hygiene, read prescription directions, and identify obstacles when walking. Similarly, hearing loss affects your ability to stay connected to the outside world, resulting in isolation and eventual cognitive impairment. With masks being common practice in healthcare settings, on a practical level, hearing-impaired seniors are no longer able to read lips.

Other Recommendations

Don't rule out extensive work due to age alone. Chronological age alone should never dictate treatment. Patients and dentists must take into account the patient's overall health and individual circumstances and, for many seniors, what's really important is a good meal. My mother-in-law, at age eighty, bemoaned that she had trouble eating nuts. She had been a very successful denture wearer and up until that point could eat whatever she wanted. With her advanced age, I was initially hesitant to perform invasive dental work, but we ultimately placed two implants to improve the stability of her lower denture. This treatment increased her quality of life immensely and gave her the ability to eat every kind of food—nuts included.

None of us knows how long we will live. Neither your biases, nor your dentist's, as in the case of my mother-in-law, should prevent you from seeking the best care. If you're healthy enough to undergo implant treatment or any other significant dental work, then it deserves serious consideration.

Don't rule out cosmetic treatment. I once had a patient who confessed he disliked his nose. All his life, it made him feel insecure. Finally, at age eighty, he decided to do something about it and got a nose job. When I saw him again months later, I honestly couldn't tell the difference. But he was thrilled—and then proceeded to ask about fixing his teeth.

Decide what's important. I've had more than one patient say wistfully, "You know, my teeth used to be my best asset." They were recalling their perfect dentition, now yellowed, jagged, and crooked. For a few of these folks, we embarked on a full cosmetic treatment because this was important to their self-image and self-esteem.

Find a dentist who will listen to you. One unfortunate by-product of age is the attitude of some healthcare providers who minimize or even disregard elderly patients' symptoms and complaints. If your dentist ignores your questions or requests, find someone else.

Treatment That Must Be Seriously Considered

You may decide that you only want to do the bare minimum to maintain your teeth. But what exactly does this mean? There are certain conditions that must be treated, or at least evaluated by a dentist.

Infection Infection can spread from your mouth to the rest of your body. As we've seen in recent years with COVID-19, in seniors with less responsive immune systems, an uncontrolled infection can escalate into a life-threatening event.

In seniors, all new infections should be treated, even ones that may be asymptomatic. One possible exception is the long-standing small, chronic infection associated with an old root canal. These infections may be dormant for years, if not decades. However, periodic X-ray evaluation is highly recommended to monitor any changes. If the infection appears to enlarge on the X-ray, it must be addressed.

Cavities   Most cavities over a certain size will grow if untreated. If your dentist suggests a filling, follow her advice. But what if the tooth already has a large filling and she says you need a crown? If you're physically and financially capable, there's no reason not to proceed.

But what if you cannot fathom the idea of two long appointments? An alternative to a crown is a silver amalgam filling. Easy-to-handle, long lasting, and affordable, amalgam is probably the most widely used material worldwide for fillings in back teeth. It's an excellent substitute when a crown cannot be done. In recent years, the popularity of amalgam has faded in favor of tooth-colored composites, which don't hold up nearly as well when used in big fillings. Some younger dentists are not even trained in the use of amalgam. Nevertheless, it's a material that has withstood the test of time.

Sometimes, seemingly overnight, patients develop multiple cavities simultaneously. Six months later, there are recurring cavities around the new fillings. It's frustrating for patient and dentist alike. In these situations, it may be unrealistic to do filling after filling when more reasonable approaches exist. Glass ionomer may be an alternative. Usually considered a temporary filling material, glass ionomer actually holds up better in certain areas than composites. It is ideal for cavities under the gum. One bonus is that glass ionomer releases fluoride into the tooth to keep the cavity in check.

Another option is silver diamine fluoride (SDF), a noninvasive, inexpensive material used to stop the progression of decay. No anesthetic or injection is required. It is effective with seniors, children, and anyone suffering from rampant tooth decay. For example, SDF would be a useful technique to manage cavities in a drug user until the patient can commit to more permanent restorations.

Tooth Breakage or Loss   What if a tooth breaks off at the gumline or falls out entirely? There's no single or right answer for this question. It depends on the tooth, the other teeth in the mouth, and the risk to the patient's health. Before her death, my mother lived in a memory care facility, and a couple of her teeth did break off at the gumline. One had an old root canal and the other probably had a nonreactive nerve. Neither seemed to cause her pain or affect her ability to eat. Because she was also non-ambulatory and suffered from advanced dementia, we decided to leave it alone. As a dentist, even though I disliked seeing the gaps, it was the right approach for her overall well-being.

In any of these situations, if it's feasible, at least get an exam to determine if there's any danger of a serious infection.

Financial Planning

We've already established that dentistry is expensive and that there is very limited coverage under Medicare. Even if Medicare were expanded to include dental coverage, chances are it would be basic in nature. Don't expect implants to be covered.

Several years prior to retirement, if you're fortunate enough to have dental insurance, create a plan with your dentist. Anticipate what specific dental work might be needed in the years ahead and proactively address these needs before you lose your dental coverage. Additionally, be sure to budget for your dental needs in retirement. Many people underestimate their healthcare expenses after retirement. Overall medical spending increases with age, with those over age eight-five facing the largest expenditures.

It's no longer assumed that you'll lose your teeth in old age. With consistent home care, a good dentist, and long-term planning, you can anticipate a lifetime of healthy function.

CHILDREN

Before your child even has teeth, his mouth should be evaluated, preferably by the pediatrician at the hospital. In addition to ruling out cleft palate, the doctor will be looking for a condition known as tongue-tie. The tongue is connected to the floor of the mouth by a ligament called the lingual frenulum. When that strand of tissue is too short, it restricts the movement of the tongue and can prevent the newborn from forming a seal with his tongue and successfully breastfeeding.

Breast versus Bottle Feeding

The decision about whether to breastfeed is a very personal one for the mother. We all know that breastfeeding transfers immunity from mother to child and may reduce some childhood allergies. But did you know that breastfeeding may also lessen the chances of future orthodontia for your child? Studies have shown that children who are exclusively breastfed for the first six months of life are less likely to manifest overbites, crossbites, or open bites.[4] In overbites, the front upper teeth stick out excessively beyond the lower teeth. With cross-bites, the lower back teeth jut out past the upper back teeth; the reverse, where the upper teeth extend and cover part of the lower teeth, is normal. In open bites, the top and bottom teeth, usually the front ones, don't meet together when the mouth is closed. I once had a patient, the mother of a three-year-old, recount her frustrating experience. As an infant, her daughter had great difficulty mastering breastfeeding. The mother consulted with the pediatrician and a lactation specialist. Nothing worked, and her baby was losing weight, officially diagnosed with "failure to thrive." This went on for much longer than necessary before the mother finally switched pediatricians. Her new physician recognized the problem immediately—the baby suffered from tongue-tie. It was impossible for her to form the seal required for breastfeeding, much less latch onto the breast.

The treatment is surprisingly simple: Snip the frenulum and free the tongue's range of motion. In this case, because the condition had gone on for so long, the child had to learn how to use her tongue to successfully feed. Although her daughter is now a normal, healthy toddler, this ordeal could've been avoided.

The Role of Fluoride

Fluoride is absorbed into the body in two ways: systemically and topically. When fluoride is ingested, it is incorporated into the enamel matrix of developing permanent teeth to strengthen them. In fully formed teeth, the fluoride ions are exchanged for the hydroxyl ions in the existing enamel matrix. While less effective, this topical method—via fluoride varnishes, gels, toothpaste, and mouthwash—does offer protection against cavities.

Fluoride was discovered accidentally. When a young dentist named Frederick McKay opened a practice in Colorado Springs in the early 1900s, he was shocked to find that many of his patients had teeth with a color that resembled chocolate. McKay enticed G. V. Black, a renowned dental researcher, to take a look. Although the two were unable to pinpoint a cause, they soon realized that these mottled teeth were resistant to decay. He began suspecting a link to the water supply, and it would take him thirty years to show that high levels of naturally occurring fluoride in the water were responsible for both the cavity protection and the discoloration.[5]

In 1945—almost fifty years later—Grand Rapids, Michigan, became the first city in the world to fluoridate its drinking water. The rate of cavities dropped by 60 percent in newly developing teeth.[6]

When fluoride is added at an ideal 1 part per million (ppm), the teeth do not discolor but become stronger and more resistant to decay. Today, 75 percent of Americans served by public water systems receive fluoride. The Centers for Disease Control and Prevention (CDC) considers this one of the top-ten public health achievements of the twentieth century. With the predominance of fluoride in consumer dental products, the amount added to drinking water has been revised to 0.7 ppm.[7] Fluoridated water is even available through bottled water vendors.

In late 2020, a new fluoridation tablet system was approved. Hailed as the first fluoride technology advancement in decades, this system promises to be more cost effective. It will provide smaller communities without the budget or infrastructure to incorporate fluoride into their drinking water.

Despite widespread use and proven benefits, fluoride has been mired in controversy. Detractors claim it is a neurotoxin, resulting in lower IQ scores in children. It should be noted that some of the studies used to support this claim were conducted in areas with excessively high naturally occurring fluoride. Others object on the basis of individual freedom yet make no mention of the chlorine added to drinking water as a disinfectant. Still others debunk its efficacy. Nevertheless, until we can ensure dental care for every child, fluoride remains the single most effective means of reducing dental disease.

The Primary Teeth

There are twenty primary teeth in total, ten in each arch. These arches, upper and lower, consist of four molars in the back (two on each side), and six incisors in the front, including the two canines, one on each side in front of the molars. Usually the lower front teeth are the first to erupt at around five months of age. By age two, most children have all twenty teeth. Delays in eruption are not cause for concern; rarely are baby teeth congenitally missing.

When the first permanent tooth erupts, parents often ask why it's so yellow. It's not that the permanent tooth is yellow; it's that the baby teeth around it, with their greater concentration of enamel, are so white.

If there are spaces between the teeth, be grateful. This indicates that there may be sufficient room to accommodate all the permanent teeth. When there is crowding of the baby teeth, I warn parents to start an orthodontic fund. Almost always, their child will need braces.

The Permanent Teeth

Including the wisdom teeth (third molars), there are thirty-two permanent teeth, sixteen in each arch. Each arch has six molars, three on each side, in the back. Preceding the molars are the four premolars (or bicuspids), two on each side. In front of them are the six incisors, identical to the pattern found in the primary dentition—the canine (or cuspid), the lateral incisor, and the central incisor (front tooth). Beginning from the back of the mouth, the sequence is as follows: third molar, second molar, first molar, second premolar, first premolar, canine, lateral incisor, central incisor.

The lower central incisors are usually the first to erupt, around age five. These are followed by the first molars, which are, for obvious reasons, also referred to as the six-year molars. Next are the central incisors, at age seven or eight, then the lateral incisors, at around age eight or nine. The period from ages nine to twelve represents a busy time of change, culminating with the appearance of the second molars, also called the twelve-year molars. By this time, the remainder of the baby teeth will have loosened and fallen out, replaced by their permanent counterparts. Much later, between the ages of sixteen and twenty-five, the third molars erupt. When there is insufficient room, they remain impacted in the mouth.

These dates are guidelines, and parents shouldn't be too concerned if there are delays. Sometimes delays are caused because there's simply not enough room for the permanent tooth to erupt. A prematurely extracted baby tooth usually results in delayed eruption of the corresponding permanent tooth. Prolonged delays should be checked out with an X-ray, as the permanent tooth may be congenitally missing. Aside from wisdom teeth, the upper lateral incisor and the lower premolars are the most commonly missing teeth. Occasionally, instead of being absent, the lateral presents itself as smaller and incompletely formed, and is called a peg lateral. Congenitally missing teeth and peg laterals may have a genetic component, as they're often evident within families.

The First Dental Visit

Both the American Dental Association and the Academy of Pediatric Dentistry recommend that your child's first dental visit should take place after that first tooth appears, but no later than the first birthday. One reason given for this recommendation is so that your child can get accustomed to going to the dentist and view it as a positive experience. I can still recall my own children's early experiences at the pediatrician. They were anything but positive. Each visit usually meant one vaccine injection or another. Try to picture your child sitting in a dental chair and opening his mouth for an extended period of time. At age one or two, even five minutes is an ambitious goal.

The other reason is to catch any emerging conditions early. As the tongue-tie example above indicates, this is important. Either your dentist or a knowledgeable pediatrician needs to examine your baby's mouth. With my children, this occurred during their periodic pediatrician appointments. If you prefer to have a dentist examine your child, the visit should take no more than a few minutes. What's the ideal time for a dedicated dental visit that engages your child? I recommend waiting until age three.

The decision whether to take your child to your family dentist or a pediatric dentist will depend on two factors. First, does your family dentist like treating children? Doing a procedure such as a filling on a fully awake child is part short-order cook and part circus clown. The dentist must work quickly and efficiently while entertaining and distracting the patient. He may prefer to spend his time doing crowns, veneers, or adult fillings. Not only are these procedures more profitable, but he can take his time and create restorations he'll be proud of. If he does enjoy treating children, it may be more convenient to have the same dentist for the entire family. Checkup appointments can be scheduled together, and your dentist will have an opportunity to bond with the family. One of my most rewarding professional memories is seeing patients I treated as three-year-olds grow into independent adults. I considered it a gift to be a part of their lives.

Second, you know your child best. Does she require more time? Are there any special needs that would be better served by a pediatric dentist? Have a frank discussion with your dentist. He can probably provide vetted referrals.

What Happens during the First Visit? With a first adult dental appointment, there are understood goals: examination, including necessary X-rays, diagnosis, and cleaning, and a discussion of the findings and any recommended treatment. The child visit is much more fluid—and dependent on your child.

In my practice, an ideal visit began with giving the child a ride in the dental chair. Then we used the intraoral camera to take a photo of the child and display it on the screen. I explained that this camera could also take pictures of his teeth. Next, I showed him the instruments and tools, beginning with the mirror that goes into the mouth. I handed him the mirror and let him feel it. I took the "tooth counter"—an explorer with a sharp tip—and touched my gloved fingernail to show the child it doesn't hurt. I introduced him to "Mr. Thirsty," the suction that may also invade his mouth. I ended the demonstration with the polisher and invited him to try one of the "toothpastes," or polishing pastes. I asked him to guess how many teeth he has and told him we would count them.

If this part went well, I reclined the dental chair and proceeded to examine his teeth. I counted as I did this, to fulfill the promise and to distract him. Simultaneously I was also checking his mouth for anything unusual and evaluating his hygiene. I finished with the polishing, calling it "tickling his teeth." While my assistant engaged the patient with "Mr. Thirsty" drinking a cup of water and making him a balloon out of a glove, I talked to the parent about the findings and recommendations. The child then left with a printed picture of himself or his teeth, a brush, and a toy.

Ideally, this visit gave me a chance to evaluate the child's mouth for any developmental issues. Sometimes there were abnormalities or brewing cavities that required further investigation. Often, even at this young age, there were bite irregularities where early intervention might eliminate the need for future braces.

The majority of three-year-olds participate in this ritual enthusiastically. But if the child is reluctant throughout any of this, the dentist shouldn't force the situation. Some children dislike the rotary polisher. Others need to be on their mother's lap. Still others refuse to open their mouths, in which case, the appointment can be postponed for three to six months before trying again. The key is for your child to have a positive experience. It's important for both the dentist and the parent to have patience.

Part of the first appointment involves interacting with the parents and gathering information. In addition to asking the parents about diet and hygiene, information concerning oral habits such as thumb sucking, sleep quality and mouth breathing, and fluoride consumption can direct and individualize the conversation for their child. It assists the dentist in sharing relevant information. Many parents, especially if this is their first child, can benefit from their dentist's expertise and knowledge.

When my brother was a preschooler, he had cavities on his upper front teeth, the result of going to sleep each night with a bottle of grape juice, a condition referred to as bottle caries. My parents simply didn't realize the juice would pool for hours around his teeth and rot them beyond repair. For years, my brother walked around without his four upper front teeth, and he was prominently cast during the school holiday programs when they sang "All I Want for Christmas Is My Two Front Teeth."

You may have noticed that I have not mentioned a cleaning or X-rays. Children rarely form tartar. Apart from some stains, there's not much to clean. Therefore, the examination is really the critical part of the routine appointment. At this young age, taking an X-ray may be the most traumatic part of the visit. X-rays should be taken only if a problem is suspected. Many young children have spaces in between their back teeth, making visual examination of these cavity-prone areas easy to do. If an X-ray is required, sometimes the parent will be asked to remain in the room to hold the X-ray in position rather than risking multiple unreadable X-rays. It's unreasonable to expect dental office personnel to habitually perform this task—recall Dr. Kells, who developed cancer in his hands from repeated and prolonged exposure to X-rays.

Recommendations for Home Care

In many TV shows and movies, a parent invariably tells a child as young as three to "go upstairs, get ready for bed, and brush your teeth." But young children need hands-on assistance; parental consistency and involvement are critical.

- *Diet:* Children seem to love sugar, and it would be unrealistic to deprive them of it entirely. Follow the guidelines in chapter 8 regarding the consumption of sugar. Additionally, make sure your child consumes enough calcium, found in dairy products and many vegetables such as broccoli and sweet potatoes. Adequate calcium is required for the development of strong bones and teeth.
- *Hygiene:* Teeth should be cleaned as soon as they develop. Six-month-old infants generally get fed before bedtime. It's important to wipe the teeth with a washcloth or finger cloth after your baby ingests breast milk or formula. If possible, to avoid bottle caries, stick to water only just before bed. As a general rule, children under the age of ten cannot properly brush their teeth. Allow them to brush by themselves, but follow up with parental brushing, especially before bedtime. To encourage more effective brushing, pink disclosing tablets can be used.

Available in drugstores, when chewed, these tablets will dye teeth pink in plaque-covered areas that need further brushing. Once your child can see the "dirty" areas, he'll be able to brush better. And although your preteen will likely balk, all children need help with flossing.

- *Fluoride:* Check the CDC website (https://nccd.cdc.gov/doh _mwf/default/default.aspx) to see if your local water is fluoridated. If it isn't, consider getting fluoridated bottled water. Permanent teeth begin calcifying at birth, and the process continues until the preteen years (with the exception of the wisdom teeth, which form later). Fluoride incorporated into the developing enamel will make these teeth more resistant to decay. As for brushing with fluoridated toothpaste, the ADA recommends smearing a layer of fluoridated toothpaste on the teeth of infants and toddlers. A more conservative approach may be to skip the fluoridated toothpaste until you're confident your child can spit out the excess rather than swallowing it. As your child ages, a pea-sized allotment of toothpaste is recommended.

- *Thumb/finger sucking or pacifier use:* The finger or pacifier creates force that can make the palate higher and narrower, resulting in a narrower upper jaw. It can also cause the upper jaw to elongate, leaving an open bite in the front. Moreover, the finger or pacifier pushes the tongue toward the floor of the mouth instead of the tip of the tongue resting naturally and passively at the palate behind the front teeth. Besides altering the bite, prolonged finger sucking or pacifier use can lead to a cascading series of consequences including tongue thrusting, mouth breathing, sleep disturbances, and focus and concentration issues. To prevent permanent changes in the jaws and the bite, this habit should be eliminated by the age of four or five.

Recommendations for Professional Care

Parents can introduce their child to the importance of good lifelong dental care. When these practices begin in childhood, patients are likely to continue such habits into adulthood. More than once, a patient has said to me, "I'm here because I promised my mother I would take care of my teeth."

- See a dentist every six months. Between the time the first permanent tooth appears until the eruption of the second molar, an exam every six months is ideal, if for no other reason than to monitor the progress of oral development. For the average child, that encompasses ages five or six through ages twelve or thirteen. If your preteen has braces, a cleaning every three months is highly advisable.

  Sealants are coatings placed on the chewing surface of newly erupted permanent molars to prevent cavities. In cavity-prone children, sealants can also be applied to the premolars. This is a cost effective, noninvasive method of preventing cavities, but it is important to understand that sealants cannot prevent cavities that form elsewhere on the tooth, most commonly in between two teeth. In order for the sealant to be successful, the tooth must be kept dry during the procedure. This is more challenging than it would first appear, especially with little six-year-old boys, who tend to gag. Postpone the sealants until the child is older if saliva control is an obstacle. Adult patients have told me over the years that their previous dentist recommended sealants for their unfilled molars. If you've reached age thirty without a cavity on the chewing surface, you don't need a sealant.

  After the cleaning, children may receive a fluoride treatment, either annually or semiannually, depending on dental insurance coverage. The goopy trays of years past—which had to remain inserted for several minutes and often induced gagging—have been replaced by fluoride varnishes that are painted on in a matter of seconds and left to air-dry. It is another simple, cost-effective method of prevention. There may come a day when fluoride varnishes will be purchased directly by the consumer with instructions on how to apply it to your children.

Your Child Needs Fillings (Gasp!)

Often, when parents are told their child needs a filling, they will say, "But it's only a baby tooth." But just like in the permanent teeth, a cavity in a baby tooth can enlarge to the point where it triggers acute pain and infection. The pulp in a primary tooth is larger in proportion to the tooth and closer to the surface, so negative outcomes can occur much faster. Infections or abscesses that result can harm the developing permanent teeth. To spare your child unnecessary pain or discomfort, and to avoid damaging the permanent teeth, the baby tooth needs to be treated.

There are several possible courses of action:

- A composite resin filling can be placed. For children with developing brains and neural systems, silver amalgam should be avoided.
- If the cavity is large and the tooth is already loose, extracting the tooth rather than filling it makes sense.
- If the cavity is large and the tooth is extremely loose, let it fall out on its own.
- With a smaller cavity, while no one can predict its progression, your dentist can make an educated guess whether the tooth will fall out on its own before the cavity becomes problematic. If that is the case, watchful waiting may be the solution.
- Lastly, SDF can arrest the cavity. One benefit to SDF is that it doesn't require an injection of local anesthetic, making it a good interim solution for very young children. The one drawback is its unsightly dark color, making it appear that a cavity might still be present.

Your Child Needs Anesthetic for the Filling   With a filling or extraction, your child will almost always get a shot of local anesthetic. Dentists are experts at giving relatively pain-free injections. Some of the most phobic patients I've encountered are ones who had work done without anesthetic when they were children. More than one person has recalled their childhood dentist saying, "Oh, it's only a baby tooth. It won't hurt." This is patently false—and a disservice to the child.

Nitrous oxide, also known as laughing gas, is a useful adjunct in treating children. It relaxes the child and allows him to remain still longer. It is extremely safe and doesn't linger in the body afterward. Perhaps your child has multiple cavities, some of which may involve a pulpotomy (a child's root canal where the top portion of the pulp is removed), followed by a preformed crown . Or maybe you have a child with special needs. Being sedated may be the best way to treat your child with the least trauma. A dental anesthesiologist may be brought in by your general dentist to administer and oversee this process, just as you would find in a hospital procedure with the surgeon and anesthesiologist. Pediatric dentists and oral surgeons are also trained in sedation techniques.

Tips for Parents

- Stay out of the treatment room. Except in very rare cases, your child will tolerate the procedure better if you wait in the reception area.
- Send a favorite stuffed animal or toy or similar object for your child to hold. Also consider sending headsets and favorite stories or music.
- Depending on the type of anesthesia, restrict your child's eating prior to the procedure or limit it to a light snack.
- After the procedure, refrain from excessively praising your child or promising a reward. If you treat this appointment as a normal occurrence, your child will learn to view it as such. Making a fuss only sends the message to your child that this is a big deal and an unpleasant experience.

Your Child Snores as Loudly as Your Spouse

Everyone snores occasionally, but unexplained loud snoring in children is not normal. Approximately 10 to 12 percent of children snore occasionally. It's estimated that 1.2 to 5.7 percent of these children suffer from obstructive sleep apnea, a condition that may impact them adversely for the rest of their lives.[8] Obstructive sleep apnea can cause impaired cognitive development, behavior issues, poor academic performance, and even high blood pressure.

Sometimes loud snoring stems from a too-small mouth, crowded teeth, a large tongue or tonsils, or a narrow airway. A trained dentist is in the perfect position to check for this condition, since she is already examining your child's mouth. While she may not be the one to treat the problem, she can refer your child to the appropriate medical provider, such as an orthodontist to expand the jaws and create more space for the teeth and tongue. By catching this early, the dentist has provided an invaluable service.

The reasons for snoring are varied. Your child's tonsils and adenoids, which reside in the back of the throat, may be unusually large or may become swollen as a result of infection, blocking the airway and causing snoring. A cold, allergies, or asthma attack can cause congestion that leads to snoring. Just like adults, markedly overweight children have a greater tendency to snore. Any obstruction that affects a child's ability to breathe through the nose, such as a deviated septum, can result in mouth breathing and snoring. Finally, environmental factors such as poor air quality or secondhand smoke can cause snoring.

You may not even be aware your child is snoring unless you're sleeping in the same room. Here are some signs that may suggest your toddler or young child is pathologically snoring:

- Sleeping with the mouth open, head tilted, and/or neck outstretched
- Gasping while sleeping
- An inability to fully close the mouth in resting position
- Nose frequently clogged
- Lips dry, cracks forming at the corner of the lips (angular chelitis)
- Teeth grinding

In older children, additionally be on the lookout for:

- Morning headaches
- Excessive daytime sleepiness
- Difficulty focusing in school, with a possible diagnosis of attention deficit hyperactivity disorder (ADHD)
- Bed-wetting
- Obesity

Pathological snoring may also be an indication of sleep-disordered breathing or sleep apnea. A 2019 YouTube video, "Finding Connor Deegan," details one boy's story about behavior issues and learning disorders where the root cause was found to be sleep apnea.[9]

In simple terms, Connor was not getting enough oxygen to his brain because of his small mouth and narrow, limited airway. Once that was corrected, his life changed for the better. While this may not be the case with your snoring child, the situation does warrant further investigation and follow-up with a medical professional.

A complete evaluation includes a physical examination of the airway anatomy, including the tonsils, adenoids, uvula, tongue, and any physical nasal obstructions. X-ray evaluation of the upper and lower jaws and airway is necessary, as is a sleep study. A functional evaluation of tongue position and habits such as teeth grinding is useful. A video of the child sleeping may be helpful.

A thorough study will likely involve doctors from different disciplines, including ear-nose-throat physicians, pediatricians, dentists, and speech therapists. Some orthodontists and pediatric dentists are trained to treat these issues. The problem is that not all doctors are trained adequately in this area; unless they seek out additional training, general dentists don't receive sufficient education in sleep-disordered breathing. When faced with a diagnosis of ADHD, it can be frustrating for parents to find guidance with the appropriate healthcare providers. But as Connor Deegan's story proves, there are knowledgeable doctors out there who can help.

Depending on the examination findings, treatment may include:

- Orthodontic expansion of the jaws, a standard orthodontic practice that is easy and well tolerated by young patients
- Other orthodontic functional appliances to guide jaw growth
- Removal of the tonsils and/or adenoids
- Medication or environmental changes to manage allergies
- Correction of nasal obstructions such as a deviated septum
- Chiropractic body manipulations
- Sleep hygiene education

Preteens and Adolescents

This is a challenging period of life, both for the teen and the parents. While no teen wants to be the only kid on the team wearing a mouth guard or subjected to yet another vaccine, the steps parents take at this stage will benefit their child later in life.

Athletic Mouth Guards   Countless adults end up with ugly crowns on a front tooth, the result of a childhood accident. Whether it's a team sport or skateboarding in the neighborhood, a mouth guard is a great idea. It will act as a shock absorber in a fall and prevent a permanent tooth from breaking or getting knocked out.

Options range from custom made to the store-bought boil-and-fit variety. Occasionally a dentist/parent will make mouth guards for their child's entire team or a neighborhood dentist will do so as part of a marketing campaign.

HPV Vaccine   The human papillomavirus (HPV) causes nine out of every ten cases of cervical cancer. In the United States, HPV is responsible for 70 percent of oropharyngeal cancers, those located in the back of the throat.[10] Due to their not easily accessible locations, these cancers are difficult to visualize and diagnose. HPV is also a cause of cervical warts.

None of us wants to imagine our preteen engaging in sexual activity, but the reality is that oral sex is occurring at earlier and earlier ages. When they were introduced in 2006, HPV vaccines were administered to high school girls and young women only. This was shortly broadened to include boys. Now HPV vaccines are recommended for preteens at age eleven or twelve and can be given as early as age nine. I routinely discussed this with the parents of this age group, sometimes to horrified reactions. Nevertheless, it's a topic that every dentist who treats children should be bringing up.

Bleaching   The interest in bleaching seems to be coming from younger and younger patients. I have had elementary school children ask to whiten their teeth. Although this is obviously a family decision, I worry about this emphasis on physical beauty in a world where twenty-year-olds are getting "preventive" Botox for future wrinkles and where data indicate that the artificially beautiful images on social media adversely affect the self-esteem and mental health of young people.

The bleaching itself isn't harmful. The implication that teeth *need* to be bleached is.

It may seem odd to lump children and seniors in the same chapter, but they do share one thing in common: Both groups have unique characteristics and require oversight and special care. As a society, how we treat our youth and elderly represents, respectively, our hope for the future and our respect for the past.

13

SPECIALIST REFERRALS—WHY CAN'T YOU JUST DO IT, DOC?

When they were not cutting hair or giving shaves, barbers used to double as dentists, extracting infected teeth. They weren't formally trained in the medical field, but barbers did possess the requisite sharp tools. It wasn't until 1723 that Pierre Fauchard, a French surgeon widely considered the father of modern dentistry, published the first book detailing the comprehensive practice of dentistry. In the late 1700s, Paul Revere advertised his services as a dentist in a Boston newspaper. A silversmith by trade, Revere was also an artist and a successful businessman. Dentistry, it seemed, was a side gig; certainly, there were no dental specialists.

In 1930, specialization in dentistry began with the creation of the American Board of Orthodontics, the world's first dental specialty organization. Today there are twelve dental specialties recognized by the American Dental Association. As of 2021, more than 21 percent of the almost 202,000 dentists in the United States were specialists.[1] This trend toward specialization is evident across the medical field. I recently took my dad to the ophthalmologist. The doctor walked into the room and said, "You know, I'm a retinologist, not a glaucoma specialist, but I'll see you *this* time."

So what constitutes a dental specialty? It must meet the following requirements:

- The specialty must have a sponsoring organization.
- It must require a unique and advanced set of knowledge and skills.
- A minimum of two years of additional training is required for a dentist to become a specialist.
- It must benefit patients.
- It must prove scientifically that it contributes new knowledge and research opportunities to dentistry.

TYPES OF DENTAL SPECIALTIES

Some of these specialties, such as orthodontics, are familiar to everyone. Others you may never have heard of, but all specialists have this in common: Besides completing the mandatory years of additional training, many specialists are board certified in their particular area. Board certification involves successfully passing examinations that demonstrate the individual's knowledge.

In general, specialists earn more money than general dentists. Before the COVID-19 pandemic, general dentists made, on average, 60 percent of a specialist's net income. By 2020, general dentists were only making 53 percent compared to specialists.[2]

- *Dental anesthesiology:* Some patients are so anxious they cannot tolerate a procedure even with laughing gas or medication. The dental anesthesiologist sedates the patient and monitors the entire procedure from beginning to end.
- *Dental public health:* Dental public health specialists deal with communities in the education, prevention, and control of dental disease. Almost all states have a dental director who works with the entire public health team.[3] As we have seen in the recent COVID-19 pandemic, this coordination of effort can be critical for effective public health measures.

- *Endodontics:* Endodontists do root canals and other procedures associated with the dental pulp.
- *Oral and maxillofacial pathology:* If you have a suspicious growth in your mouth that requires a biopsy, the pathologist is the specialist who renders an opinion on the lesion. It's likely you will never meet the pathologist or even know his identity. Pathologists are frequently dental school faculty.
- *Oral and maxillofacial radiology:* Radiologists are also not generally known to patients. Most likely your scan or X-ray will be sent to the radiologist for a written evaluation. Like the pathologists, these specialists are also typically affiliated with dental schools.
- *Oral and maxillofacial surgery:* You might see an oral and maxillofacial surgeon to have the biopsy done. These specialists also place implants, take out wisdom teeth, fix broken jaws, and perform all other surgery related to the mouth and jaw area. This specialty requires another four to six years of training after dental school, and most finish their programs with an MD degree as well.
- *Oral medicine:* You may be referred to an oral medicine specialist if you have a medially complex situation, one that stumps your general dentist.
- *Orofacial pain:* Sometimes despite examination and testing, the source of pain remains elusive. Or perhaps you suffer from chronic pain around the mouth and jaw area. An orofacial pain specialist may be able to help.
- *Orthodontics and dentofacial orthopedics:* Everyone knows what an orthodontist does, but did you know that this specialist also treats skeletal abnormalities of the jaws and face?
- *Pediatric dentistry:* The pediatric dentist takes care of patients from infancy through adolescence.
- *Periodontics:* The periodontist treats the supporting structures of the teeth: the gums. They also place implants and extract the occasional tooth.
- *Prosthodontics:* You may see a prosthodontist if your mouth needs extensive restoration and rehabilitation. Usually these are complex cases.

Notice what's missing from this list:

- *Cosmetic dentistry:* Any dentist can call himself a cosmetic dentist, and many do. There are multiple organizations with either "Cosmetic Dentistry" or "Aesthetic Dentistry" in their names that provide dentists with opportunities for education and collaboration.
- *Implant dentistry:* Similarly, any dentist can claim to specialize in implant dentistry, even though no such specialty currently exists. There are organizations that focus on the field of implants. Some of these organizations have successfully sued state dental boards to allow their members to advertise their implant credentials, knowledge, and expertise.
- *Dental sleep medicine:* While organizations exist that specifically focus on sleep apnea and sleep medicine, it is not a recognized dental specialty.

HOW DOES YOUR DENTIST DECIDE ON THE PARTICULAR SPECIALIST?

Patients may decide they need a specialist and choose one themselves. For example, your neighbor raves about her child's orthodontist, and even though your own dentist hasn't mentioned anything about your son's crooked teeth, you think it's time for a consultation and make an appointment. Most referrals, though, originate from the general dentist, and it is not uncommon for them to give patients more than one name and leave the ultimate decision to them. Dentists may refer particular specialists for a variety of reasons:

- They may have existing working relationships. Almost all general dentists have experience and collaborative relationships with specialists such as orthodontists, oral surgeons, periodontists, and endodontists. Often they have "go-to" specialists with whom they've worked for years. They have seen those specialists' work and evaluated their clinical skills and expertise.

- They may know each other personally. Chances are they met while in dental school, or at a professional function such as a continuing education course or a community outreach event. Maybe the specialist is just beginning his career and introduced himself recently. Perhaps they know each other socially. Maybe they're golfing buddies.
- Your dentist may pick a specialist from an insurance list. Depending on the type of insurance you have (discussed in chapter 3), there may be restrictions on which specialist you can see. While you are certainly free to choose any doctor you wish, if a particular specialist is not part of your insurance plan, the services may be more costly or may not be covered. There's also a possibility your dentist might not recognize any of the specialists on the insurance list.
- The specialist may work in your dentist's office. With rising office overhead, not all specialists want an office of their own. Itinerant specialists may work with multiple dentists, traveling on a schedule to each office to service patients. This arrangement benefits your dentist by allowing her to keep some of the revenue in-house. The advantage to you is convenience and familiarity. You don't have to figure out the logistics of a new location. However, the disadvantage is twofold. First, the specialist will be less accessible; should a complication arise, your general dentist will likely be managing it since the specialist may only be available periodically or on a predetermined schedule. The other disadvantage is a lack of choice: You're limited to one option, and there may be subtle pressure for you to go with your dentist's recommendation.

Depending on the connection, your general dentist may not have seen the specialist's work firsthand. He may or may not have direct knowledge of the specialist's clinical skills. It's possible he's only familiar with the specialist's credentials or reputation, or the specialist "seems like a nice guy." Depending on the specialty, it can take a while to evaluate the results. For example, when I refer a patient to an orthodontist, it may be a couple years before I'm able to accurately access the quality of the work. However, if I send a patient for a root canal, I'll have a good idea of the specialist's skill within a relatively short time.

Don't be afraid to ask your dentist exactly what it is he likes about the specialist. Maybe there's good communication between the two of them, so the expectations of your case are fully understood by both. Perhaps the specialist sends timely reports on the outcome of your procedure, noting anything unusual. Or there may be something unique to recommend this individual. For years I worked with an endodontist and had the opportunity to see hundreds of cases. I would tell my patients, "If I needed a root canal, I would go to this guy. In fact, I sent my husband to him."

SHARE YOUR INSIGHTS

Patient insights can provide pertinent information that helps dentists decide whether to recommend a particular specialist. By all means, provide this valuable feedback about your experience to your dentist.

- What is the doctor's chairside manner like? Does he take time to answer your questions? Does he listen to you? Does he make eye contact?
- What is the front office like? Are they courteous? Efficient? How long does it take to get an appointment? Do they run on time?
- Is the office clean? Modern? How's the parking? Chances are your dentist has never actually visited the office.
- What about the financial policies? Many specialists expect to be paid up front. This is understandable since you're likely a one-time patient. Do they expect the full payment or just the portion not covered by insurance?

WHY CAN'T/WON'T YOUR DENTIST DO THE PROCEDURE?

You may be wondering, "Can't my dentist just do the extraction?" You know your dentist and have a relationship with her. There's anxiety associated with meeting a new doctor, not to mention the added inconvenience. And since the specialist's fees are higher, it'll cost you more than your regular dentist.

The simple answer is: Maybe. The decision whether to refer boils down to a judgement call, and the old adage "You don't know what you don't know" is so true. Early on in my career, I lacked the experience to anticipate what complications might occur and even the knowledge to determine which cases might be straightforward and which would be difficult. My inexperience led to some attempts where I had to subsequently contact a specialist to complete the procedure—in short, I got in over my head and had to be bailed out.

Every dentist traverses this learning curve, and there's no substitute for experience. When I finally figured out the sweet spot that incorporated my knowledge, experience, and confidence, the practice of dentistry became less stressful and more fun. Understand that your dentist may be somewhere along this continuum as well.

If the general dentist does the procedure, he is expected to perform it with the same standard of care to which specialists are held. Training and experience in specialty fields vary among general dentists. For many years I was involved with the California Dental Association peer review program, a forum for patient grievances and conflict resolution between patients and dentists. We handled a slew of Invisalign-related complaints against general dentists. Without sufficient training in the area of orthodontics, many of these general dentists were ill prepared and assumed the entry into Invisalign treatment would be easy and smooth. There are general dentists who complete extensive Invisalign training and have successfully treated thousands of patients, and if your dentist is one of them, treatment may be comparable to what you would receive from an orthodontist. The key is in identifying the qualifications of your general dentist.

There are several reasons your dentist may wish to refer you:

- The procedure is beyond the scope of their expertise. If your dentist tells you, "Trust me. You'll be in better hands with Dr. Specialist," listen to that recommendation. Don't put your dentist in the awkward position of performing a procedure he doesn't feel comfortable doing just so he won't disappoint you. Ultimately, you may both regret this.

- There are patient-related issues. For example, you may not be able to open your mouth very wide or for an extended period of time. Your general dentist may conclude that the specialist can finish the procedure in less time so that you'll be more comfortable.
- Your dentist just doesn't like doing that type of procedure. I know many dentists who don't enjoy doing root canals or dentures. It doesn't mean they're incapable of doing a satisfactory job. They may simply wish to focus their practice efforts elsewhere.

If your dentist chooses to perform the procedure herself, she must feel confident and qualified. Perhaps the case is straightforward and easy. In the realm of root canals, almost every general dentist would proceed with a root canal on an upper front tooth (central incisor) but some will refer out a lower front tooth, which contains more anatomic variation and may include two canals. Specialists almost always end up treating the more complex and difficult cases.

Perhaps the dentist has had additional training in a particular area. He may be very interested in, say, veneers, and has taken multiple hands-on courses. (I was drawn to the subject of sleep apnea and took a months-long mini-residency on the topic.) However, if you sense that your dentist is doing the procedure because she needs the business, ask for a referral.

QUESTIONS TO ASK

To determine whether you should be seeing a specialist or having your general dentist perform the procedure, consider asking the following questions to your general dentist and about the specialist:

- How many of these procedures do you do annually?
- What kind of additional training have you undertaken?
- Do you anticipate any complications, and if so, what are they?
- Do you use the same equipment a specialist would employ?
- Do you feel comfortable and confident performing this procedure?

- Would you feel equally comfortable and confident performing this procedure on a family member?
- Do you have existing relationships with specialists in the community?
- Have you any direct experience with the specialists you're recommending?
- What do you like about this particular specialist?
- If your dentist is recommending an in-house specialist: How often is the specialist physically in the office? Who will manage complications or emergencies?

Remember that there are no hard-and-fast rules about whether you should see a specialist rather than your general dentist. Each situation is different. The challenge for both patient and dentist is in arriving at the right solution most of the time.

(14)

ORTHODONTIC SECRETS

Did you know that nine out of ten people have malocclusion, literally translated as "bad bite"?[1] Of this group, it's estimated that more than half will require some kind of orthodontic treatment.[2] Braces have become so commonplace in certain communities that they are almost a rite of passage. No wonder orthodontists represent one of the highest earning dental specialties.

Fossil records indicate that when humans roamed the earth as hunter-gatherers two million years ago, they didn't suffer from malocclusion. Not only did they have straight teeth, they also had ample room for their wisdom teeth. Humans had large, powerful jaws they used to tear meat. So what happened? Our teeth remained the same, but our jaws began to shrink.

Several events contributed to this evolution. The use of stone tools allowed humans to manipulate and cut meat into bite-sized pieces, thus reducing our chewing effort. We transitioned into an agrarian society, growing a variety of softer foods to supplement our carnivorous diet. The harnessing of fire, possibly four hundred thousand years ago, meant we could cook our food into an even more manageable texture. With each of these revolutionary events in human development, our jaws continued to shrink.

Today, our diet starts with mushy baby food and proceeds to a mostly soft and processed menu. This mismatch of jaw size with tooth size and quantity has led to crowded teeth, impacted wisdom teeth, and even a smaller airway. Wisdom teeth are the most commonly congenitally missing teeth in the mouth, causing some to conjecture that they may be evolving out of existence due to insufficient space.

The first evidence of orthodontia was a gold band around a tooth of an ancient Egyptian mummy, discovered in a Roman tomb in Egypt in the early 1900s. When not thinking about more important subjects, both Hippocrates and Aristotle pondered over methods to straighten teeth. But it wasn't until the 1800s that the first orthodontic appliance was introduced. Early in the twentieth century, Edward H. Angle founded the first orthodontic school in the United States. Angle also originated a system of classifying malocclusions that is used to this day.

RECENT ADVANCES IN ORTHODONTICS

Many modern advances in orthodontics are technology driven or improvements in materials that have been applied to orthodontics.

The Bracket

Prior to the bracket, a metal band had to be fitted around the circumference of each tooth in order to attach the orthodontic wire. Not only was this cumbersome, but in an already crowded mouth, room had to be created for bands around each tooth. Patients had to wear tiny rubber bands around their teeth to prepare for the metal banding. The bracket, which is attached to the front of the tooth, eliminated the need for all this. Brackets were initially made out of metal, but in the late 1980s, the first ceramic "clear" bracket was introduced, marking the beginning of more aesthetic orthodontic options. Brackets can now be custom made to fit the individual curvature of a specific tooth.

Dental Adhesives

It's no exaggeration to say that dental adhesives revolutionized dentistry. But this adhesive technology originated from a field as far removed from dentistry as outer space: The adhesive used to bond ceramic tiles onto the space shuttle was a precursor to modern dental adhesives.

Ceramic and metal brackets are bonded onto teeth for orthodontic treatment. Dental adhesives are also used to bond tooth-colored composite fillings, paving the way for the popularity of white fillings over silver amalgams.

Cone Beam Computed Tomography

Unlike two-dimensional X-rays, cone beam computed tomography (CBCT) produces a three-dimensional view of anatomical structures. With orthodontic treatment, CBCT can provide valuable information such as patient growth analysis or the exact location of an impacted tooth. CBCT, however, delivers a lot more radiation compared to the traditional panoramic X-ray. Children are especially sensitive to X-rays, with radiation risks decreasing as people get older. In 2008, only 2 percent of children received CBCT X-ray scans in the United States. By 2020, this number had increased to 16 percent.[3] As a parent, ask questions and be vigilant. Can the same diagnostic information be obtained from a lower-dose X-ray?

Implant-Assisted Orthodontic Treatment

For particularly difficult-to-move teeth, a temporary mini-implant can be used to provide leverage. It is placed into the gum and jawbone away from the teeth, usually opposite the cheek, as an anchor to assist in moving the teeth. Typically, it is harder to move teeth toward the back of the mouth (in the direction of the ear) than toward the center of the mouth (by the chin or nose). The treatment may take longer, but without the presence of the implant, this type of movement might be too difficult to attempt. Once the treatment is completed, the mini-implant is removed.

"Fast" Orthodontics

The average orthodontic treatment time is twenty-four months, but in our fast-paced, we-want-it-yesterday world, any tool that accelerates treatment time seems worthy of consideration.

Distraction osteogenesis is a surgical technique used to alter the shape of bones by cutting slits in the bone. If the upper jaw needs to be widened, for example, distraction osteogenesis can be used to accomplish this instead of the more invasive surgery that cracks and separates the entire jaw. While there are pros and cons with this technique, one of the main advantages is reduced treatment time.

Another "fast" orthodontic technique is a gadget called the vibrating appliance. Similar in appearance to an athletic mouth guard, this device pulses when inserted, theoretically stimulating cell growth around the teeth. Two commercially available devices were reviewed and it was concluded that "there is no evidence that vibrating appliances are effective in an acceleration of orthodontic treatment time."[4] Given the data, I would recommend passing on this suggestion if your orthodontist offers it.

ALIGNER ORTHODONTICS

One recent advance, aligner orthodontics, has upended traditional bracket-and-wire orthodontics. Aligner orthodontics refers to treatment that is rendered through a series of stiff, semitransparent trays meant to be worn as many as twenty-two hours daily. This near-constant pressure on the teeth results in gradual movement.

Aligner orthodontics were first conceptualized in the early twentieth century. Mostly academic in nature, these concepts weren't translated into widespread practical or commercial use until the 1990s, when two Stanford MBA students, Zia Chishti and Kelsey Wirth, started Align Technology with their patented Invisalign system. Frustrated with his own orthodontic treatment, Chishti envisioned a CAD/CAM-designed tray system in which teeth could be moved without the use of unsightly metal brackets and wires. Initially introduced exclusively to orthodontists, Invisalign met with resistance. Align Technology then pivoted and marketed the idea to the public, spurring more than 70 percent of US orthodontists to become trained in the system.[5] The company also expanded its Invisalign offering to general dentists. In 2004, the FDA removed the restriction that Invisalign be limited to permanent teeth, thereby opening up the patient pool to include teens and preteens.

Early on, several other companies entered the aligner orthodontic arena, one of them started by one of the original Align Technology founders, who left in 2003. Litigation ensued and agreements eventually were reached. Although Align Technology dominates the marketplace, most of its patents expired in 2017 and 2019. Competitors continue to appear, hoping to capture a portion of this lucrative market.

Invisalign treatment always takes place in a dental office with treatment provided by either an orthodontist or a general dentist. Some of the newer competitors initially touted a do-it-yourself method whereby the patient would take their own impressions and the trays would arrive like an Amazon order. The company relied on the patient's word that they had X-rays and an examination prior to beginning aligner orthodontic treatment. Since then, stricter state regulations on this practice have dictated some form of professional dental oversight. As of 2020, one company, Smile Direct Club, announced it would start selling aligners through dental offices as well as online.

If you are interested in aligner orthodontics, you may be asking yourself whether you should see an orthodontist or be treated by your general dentist—who, by the way, seems eager to tackle your case. Ask your dentist how many aligner orthodontic cases she has completed successfully. The higher the number, the greater her experience with this modality. There are some general dentists who have undoubtedly done more aligner cases than their orthodontist colleagues. However, hands down, the orthodontist will know more about the subject of orthodontics. After all, he completed additional years of training in this area. The more complex the situation, the greater the need for a specialist's knowledge and expertise.

What to Watch Out for with Aligner Orthodontics

Many people, especially adults, would never have considered the "metal mouth" approach to correcting their crooked teeth.

Because of this, the introduction of aligner orthodontics revolutionized orthodontics and added an entire segment of new patients. That said, aligner orthodontics is not suitable for everyone. There are several important factors to consider.

Case Complexity   Aligner orthodontics is designed to fix simple to moderate bite problems. But what if the situation is structural and the size of the upper and lower jaw don't match? No amount of tooth movement will correct that. Or perhaps your mouth is unusually crowded, requiring treatment that involves either extracting teeth or "stripping" each tooth to narrow it in order to create the necessary space. Tray wearing alone will not accomplish this.

Compliance   To work effectively, the trays need to be worn at all times except during meals. Results will still occur with, say, ten hours of wear, but the treatment time will be longer. It's also easy to fall into the repeated habit of removing the tray prior to an important meeting or social event.

Age   Invisalign was originally intended for adults. Even adolescents with only permanent teeth were dissuaded from using Invisalign. Recently I worked at an elementary school dental screening where I saw possibly ten third-graders wearing aligner trays. This disturbed me for several reasons. First, it's hard enough to get adults to comply with the number of hours of wear required. Second, third-graders are generally poor with dental hygiene. Picture the trapped food particles residing inside the trays—and the cavities afterward. Finally, children and adolescents are constantly losing their retainers. A loss of a tray will not only add to the expense, but depending on how long it takes to replace the tray, there could be unwanted tooth movement in the interim.

Cost   In general, dentist-supervised aligner orthodontic treatment is more expensive than metal braces. The treatment includes the fee the dentist must pay for the design and fabrication of the aligner trays.

Temporomandibular Joint Changes

Some research has shown that the prolonged and continuous wearing of aligner trays causes bone density decreases in the TMJ, which may potentially affect future function.[6]

Dentist Supervised versus Do-It-Yourself

Would you extract your own tooth or perform your own skin biopsy after watching a YouTube video? As appealing as the cost savings may be, there are too many risks to proceed without direct professional supervision—and ultimately, it may end up costing you more to repair the damage. If you choose the DIY route, a thorough physical and X-ray examination is mandatory. It's not enough to have X-rays, scans, and photographs of your mouth taken somewhere and subsequently have these records reviewed remotely by a dentist or orthodontist you'll never meet. A dental professional needs to physically examine your teeth and mouth prior to starting treatment.

CURRENT TRENDS IN ORTHODONTIC TREATMENT

If it seems like every kid you see has braces, consider this: From 1996 to 2016, orthodontic spending in the United States rose by more than 70 percent, from $11.5 billion in 1996 to $19.9 billion in 2016.

The patient population is also changing. Although 75 percent of orthodontic patients are under the age of eighteen, adults are increasingly seeking treatment. In the United States, an estimated 1.61 million adults received treatment in 2018, up from 1.55 million in 2016.[7] I once had a sixty-five-year-old patient begin orthodontic treatment, paid for by her ninety-something-year-old father, who regretted not being able to provide this for his daughter when she was younger. Since adult orthodontia is primarily paid out of pocket without the benefit of any insurance assistance, it's more discretionary than orthodontic treatment for children. In my practice, several adults would ask daily about the prospect of correcting their crooked teeth. Many of them had worn braces as a child and experienced relapse of their bite. But during the Great Recession of 2007–2009, these inquiries ceased almost entirely.

The route by which patients enter orthodontic treatment has also changed. While patients are still by and large referred through their general dentists, self-referral has become more common. In recent years, with the advent of aligner orthodontics, consumers are regularly exposed to direct orthodontic advertising.

The American Association of Orthodontists recommends that every child have an orthodontic evaluation by age seven. This is sound advice because there are some problems that benefit from early intervention. But are we seeing younger and younger patients? It does appear that more and more elementary school–aged children are walking around with braces. Some of these children will eventually require a second round of treatment once they hit adolescence—in essence, a Phase I and Phase II. An additional phase of treatment naturally means greater expense, but it also means your child may have a higher likelihood of developing cavities under those metal brackets, since it's harder to brush and clean with braces.

WHEN TO BEGIN TREATMENT

In years past, orthodontic treatment didn't commence until all the permanent teeth, excluding the wisdom teeth, had erupted. If there wasn't enough room to accommodate all the teeth, then usually one or two premolars, also called bicuspids, were extracted. That's what happened to me. So is it better to start early or wait until all the permanent teeth are in?

Jaw Growth

Remember the jaws of our cavemen ancestors? The size of the jaws determines whether the teeth will be crowded. The maxilla holds the upper teeth and the mandible is home to the lower teeth. The relationship of the maxilla to the mandible may manifest in an overbite or an underbite. This usually remains stable even as the jaws grow.

Girls tend to mature physically earlier than boys, and this is reflected in their jaw growth. Between the ages of fourteen and sixteen, girls show the most jaw growth. This growth drops by half from ages sixteen to twenty.[8] As a general guideline, growth in girls usually stops two years after the onset of menstruation. Jaw growth occurs later in boys, with a spurt between ages sixteen and twenty.[9] It's not uncommon for boys to grow into their mid-twenties.

How do we know when jaw growth is complete? The most reliable method is by taking a lateral cephalometric X-ray or scan at two different points in time. If the two images are identical, it indicates a cessation of growth. For example, a scan might be taken at age twenty. If there's no discernable growth in the following year, then another scan can be taken at age twenty-one to confirm that the patient has fully matured physically.

But Wait—Something Doesn't Make Sense

Most children begin orthodontic treatment during the middle school years, around age twelve or thirteen, when all the permanent teeth except the wisdom teeth have erupted. It's safe to say that almost every preteen longs to be done with braces by the time they reach high school, and no high school senior wants to be remembered with braces in his yearbook picture, much less embark on college or a job with a mouthful of metal.

But if we wait for the permanent teeth to erupt before we start orthodontic treatment, shouldn't we also wait for the jaws to fully grow and mature? After all, once the jaws grow to their final dimensions, there may not even be a need for braces. It seems reasonable to wait for both of these elements—the eruption of teeth and the maturation of the jaws—before deciding about orthodontic treatment. Granted, there are some circumstances where beginning braces during middle school is warranted; for example, a permanent tooth may be impacted or missing, in which case a treatment plan needs to be developed early.

So, given these facts, why do we put braces on preteens?

Social Pressure   Puberty and the transition to adolescence are already an awkward and difficult time. Since the permanent teeth have erupted, it seems logical to begin orthodontic treatment in middle school. A metal mouth may be less conspicuous amid the acne, brewing hormones, and changing bodies of the early teen years. Besides, there will be resistance on the part of your high schooler if treatment is started later. I have witnessed more than one young woman break down in tears when told that her braces couldn't be removed just yet.

Control over Treatment   Orthodontic treatment requires periodic monitoring and regular appointments. While the patient is still under the direct supervision of a parent, compliance with treatment obligations will be higher. Imagine a nineteen-year-old young man living in a college environment showing up every month at the orthodontist. What are the chances of a missed or forgotten appointment?

Financial Considerations   Some insurance policies stop covering orthodontic treatment at age twenty-one. Additionally, with the financial burdens of higher education, parents may be stretched thin to pay for braces. Alternatively, if a young adult is supporting himself, he may be less inclined to budget for health expenditures once his jaw is fully mature at age twenty-five.

Unless there's an overhaul of our social constructs, it's likely that orthodontic treatment will proceed according to the same middle school timeline.

EARLY TREATMENT

What about the elementary school children who have braces or a retainer? Is this legitimate, or are we being oversold? There are specific situations where early treatment is not only desirable but highly recommended.

When Is Early Treatment Indicated?

The Crossbite   In a normal bite, the upper back teeth are positioned outside (closer to the cheek) of the lower back teeth. This means the upper jaw is wider than the lower jaw. However, if the reverse is true and the upper jaw is narrower than the lower jaw, then the child will usually shift his jaw to either left or right so that a normal bite is achieved on one side with a resultant crossbite on the opposite side.

In the maxilla, there's a suture that runs through the middle. Similar to the soft spots in a baby's skull that allows it to expand as the brain grows, this suture becomes hardened in a significant portion of girls by age eleven and boys by age fourteen.[10] Once it is fused, upper jaw growth is complete. An individual X-ray assessment can determine whether your child's suture is fused. Before the age of ten, maxilla expansion can be easily and successfully accomplished with a simple appliance.

Why fix a posterior crossbite? Not only will it lead to a more stable bite and temporomandibular joint position, but widening the upper jaw will create more space for the teeth and a more ideal airway.

The "Buck" Tooth   Does your child have a front tooth that's sticking out, just begging to be damaged in an accidental fall or athletic endeavor? It may be prudent to fix this sooner rather than later. If the child falls, breaks the tooth, and needs a root canal and crown, this dental work will need to be maintained throughout the child's life.

Snoring or Mouth Breathing   Snoring and mouth breathing are habits that may indicate a mouth that is too small or an insufficient airway. Early diagnosis and treatment will give your child a healthy start in life. Depending on the findings, treatment may involve functional appliances to manage and direct jaw growth or expansion appliances to physically widen the maxilla.

Prolonged Thumb/Finger Sucking or Pacifier Use   Beyond the age of four or five, sucking on fingers or a pacifier will result in permanent changes in the jaws. The maxilla will become narrower and the palate higher. Crowding of the permanent teeth is probable. A simple orthodontic appliance along with behavior therapy can correct this.

Missing Permanent Teeth   While there may be no actual orthodontic treatment done at an early age, an orthodontic evaluation by age seven should reveal the lack of one or more permanent teeth. One of my patients had more than a half dozen missing permanent teeth. Even though she never had braces, this early knowledge allowed us to plan for the eventual restoration of her mouth.

The lateral incisor, the tooth right beside the upper front tooth, is one of the most commonly missing teeth. From an orthodontic perspective, the decision must be made whether to move the more prominent and bulbous canine into that position or leave a space for a future implant.

These early treatment situations should be diagnosed by your general or pediatric dentist, who will then refer your child to an orthodontist if indicated. Either your dentist or the orthodontist will order the necessary diagnostic X-rays.

When Is Early Treatment Not a Good Idea?

The Underbite   An underbite occurs when the mandible protrudes beyond the maxilla. The comedian Jay Leno has an underbite. Mandibles tend to grow later than maxillas, usually in a downward and forward direction. Orthodontic treatment before the mandible has fully matured will lead to a reoccurrence of the underbite. It's prudent to wait until the child is fully grown, and with boys, this can be as late as the mid-twenties. Sometimes surgery is required in addition to braces to correct an underbite.

When It's Overtreatment   If, during the consultation, the orthodontist is introducing Phase I treatment and anticipating a Phase II treatment, be sure you understand why two phases are necessary. Sometimes two phases *are* justified. If a Phase I treatment can make the Phase II treatment significantly easier and shorter, then early treatment may be reasonable. Ask questions. Seek a second opinion and also discuss this with your general or pediatric dentist. If you're at all uncomfortable, stop and find out more. While you as the parent will not be able to determine overtreatment, seeking evaluations from other trusted professionals can assist with treatment decisions.

HOW TO HELP YOUR CHILD, PRETEEN, OR TEEN SUCCEED WITH BRACES

You may have an exceptional child, but most children and adolescents do not brush their teeth for two minutes every single time. Dental hygiene is critical with braces and clear aligners. I once examined a teenage boy who had undergone Invisalign treatment. He rarely brushed his teeth or even rinsed his mouth after eating, simply reinserting the Invisalign trays. Halfway though treatment, this patient had more than ten cavities, and the decision was made to stop his treatment. Below are some recommendations to help your child succeed with orthodontic care.

- Invest in an electric toothbrush, ideally one with a small brush head.
- To remove food particles, a water flosser is useful. Flossing aids such as floss threaders also work, but many people find them challenging and time consuming.
- Help your child eat a healthy diet.
- If headgear or elastics are involved, monitor compliance. Not using these for the recommended time will prolong treatment.
- Have your child's teeth professionally cleaned and examined every three months. I have come across many loose brackets or broken wires during these exams.
- With a busy family schedule, it's easy to lose track of orthodontist appointments. Try to be compliant.
- Once your child is finished with active orthodontic treatment, retainer use is mandatory. To quote David Sedaris in his book *Happy-Go-Lucky*, "I had braces when I was young. And when they were removed at age 17 or so, I looked fantastic. Then I ruined everything by not wearing a retainer like I was supposed to."[11]

ADULT ORTHODONTIA

Adults represent one of the fastest growing populations seeking orthodontic treatment, roughly trending with the popularity of Invisalign. What adult wouldn't find wearing a relatively transparent tray more attractive than conspicuous wires and brackets? Adults pursue orthodontic treatment for several reasons:

- Their teeth have shifted. Over a lifetime, teeth continuously move and tend to drift toward the center of the mouth. This is most evident in the crowding of the lower front teeth. As people age, these teeth become more visible—and noticeable—than the upper front teeth. Some adults who seek treatment had braces when they were young and have experienced relapse, perhaps because they weren't good about wearing a retainer. They may decide to undergo treatment again, this time with more intention and maturity.

- They needed braces as a child but never had them. Many adults who did not have braces as children decide to finally seek orthodontic treatment because they now have the financial resources to do it. Sometimes they do this alongside their teenagers, calling it a "bonding experience."
- Their dentist said it's necessary. Occasionally, restoration and rehabilitation of the dentition is impossible without moving teeth into a more strategic and ideal position. For example, cosmetic dentistry on the lower front teeth may involve moving them orthodontically to create space for the future veneers.

Before you commit to treatment, consider these factors and recommendations:

- Get an exam first. It's imperative that the teeth and mouth be healthy prior to undergoing orthodontic treatment. For adults, checking the periodontal condition is especially important. Any immediate dental concerns, such as cavities or gum problems, should be addressed before beginning orthodontic treatment.
- Brush up on your oral hygiene. Just as with children, maintaining a clean mouth during treatment will prevent dental problems later.
- Prepare to wear a retainer indefinitely. This is one of the most important questions to ask yourself: can you commit to wearing a retainer? Teeth relapse, and teeth moved during adulthood especially tend to relapse. After treatment is completed, nightly retainer use is usually recommended for one to two years. After that, you should continue wearing your retainer or your last tray approximately two to three times weekly. If you can't commit to this routine, then your time, effort, and expense will be largely wasted.
- Don't restrict yourself to aligner orthodontics. Your malocclusion may be so severe that aligner orthodontics will not correct the problem. Listen to your dentist or orthodontist. If she recommends traditional braces, resist the urge to find a practitioner who will do Invisalign. You'll definitely find someone, but it may

not be in your best interest. If you're adamant about fixing your teeth with trays, at least have a discussion with your orthodontist about how compromised the results might be and what the risks are.

- Implants will not move. Unlike teeth, which have a periodontal ligament, implants are firmly attached to the bone. Consequently, they cannot be moved orthodontically and may prevent your other teeth from moving into an ideal position. Find out beforehand if this will be a major obstacle to treatment. Involving your general dentist in this appraisal is critical; since the orthodontist doesn't do this type of dentistry, he may not be as aware of the nuances.

- Oral appliances may no longer fit. Do you have a night guard or an appliance for sleep apnea? Once orthodontic treatment begins, the appliance may no longer fit. And because your bite will be changing over time, it also doesn't make sense to fabricate a new oral appliance until the treatment is complete. If you use a sleep apnea appliance, consider switching to a CPAP machine during this period. The same caution applies to mouth guard wearers. If you're using a mouth guard to protect against nighttime grinding, the aligner tray cannot provide the same function. It is too thin and flimsy to provide the protection afforded by your mouth guard.

ORTHODONTIC CHALLENGES

There are a number of potential challenges and limitations to orthodontic work. Orthodontists understand—and routinely deal with—some of these more difficult challenges, and it is important to be aware of them.

A Stubborn Gap between Upper Front Teeth

Called a diastema, a space between the upper front teeth is easy enough to close. The difficulty is in keeping it closed. Occasionally there's a muscle attachment that interferes, which must be surgically repositioned, but sometimes the diastema reappears for no apparent reason. You can attempt to correct a diastema, or you can simply embrace it. After treatment, a wire can also be permanently bonded behind the upper front teeth to keep the space closed.

Oral Habits

Sometimes certain oral habits can cause relapse in a corrected stable bite. One is tongue thrusting, where the patient unconsciously sticks his tongue out when swallowing. Infants swallow like this, typically growing out of it by age four or five. Because we swallow approximately two thousand times each day, habitual tongue thrusting can result in an open bite, where the front teeth don't meet. Once the open bite develops, the tongue must fill in that spot during swallowing so that a seal is formed to keep liquid from leaking out—and the habit becomes reinforced. Another habit is thumb or finger sucking, which will change an orthodontically corrected bite and move teeth out of position.

These habits must be addressed and eliminated for the orthodontic treatment to be successful. For tongue thrusters, this may involve the help of a myofunctional therapist or speech therapist. For thumb suckers, there are appliances that will prevent the thumb from entering the mouth.

The Second Molars

Although these are called the twelve-year molars, they don't always fully emerge at this age. In fact, these teeth are often partially erupted or delayed in their appearance. This coincides with the time when the preteen is anticipating removal of the braces in the next year or so.

Sometimes orthodontists don't include the second molars in treatment. To be fair, it's challenging to bond a bracket onto a partially erupted second molar. But not including these critical teeth means the bite will be less than ideal, specifically when the patient moves her mouth from side to side. Long-term adverse bite changes may follow. As unappealing as this idea is to your teen, delay orthodontic completion until the second molars can be an integral part of the treatment.

Many Missing Teeth

When teeth are missing or extracted, the remaining teeth have a tendency to move into the resulting empty spaces. Excessive movement or the passage of time can result in a bite that's changed so much that it becomes almost impossible to move the teeth orthodontically back to an ideal position. Sometimes healthy teeth have to be extracted in order to restore a bite or dentition to reasonable function.

FREQUENTLY ASKED QUESTIONS

My orthodontist wants to shave some of my tooth enamel. Is that bad?

Referred to as interproximal stripping, this process involves judiciously removing some enamel on the sides of the teeth to narrow them and create more space. While everyone acknowledges that enamel is finite and precious, it boils down to simple math, really. Adding up the width of each tooth determines how much space, usually expressed in millimeters, is required in the jaw to create a straight bite. If the jaw is shorter than that, either a tooth has to be extracted or stripping must be done. The decision will depend on exactly how many millimeters of additional space is needed. Interproximal stripping will probably be carried out by your general dentist.

Who decides when orthodontic treatment is complete?

I once had a teenage patient who took a pair of pliers and removed her braces herself. She was done! In an ideal situation, though, the decision to end orthodontic treatment is a collaborative effort between your orthodontist and general dentist. The orthodontist may consider the case finished, but the general dentist may view it from a slightly different perspective. For example, if a lateral incisor is missing in the upper front area, the plan may be to leave a gap open for a future implant. The orthodontist may have accomplished this, but if the general dentist notices that the space is too narrow to accommodate the smallest implant, the space has to be made wider.

Don't be afraid to ask your general dentist to examine the bite prior to braces removal. Each professional brings a different knowledge base.

Can my night guard double as a retainer?

Absolutely. Again, some coordination and communication must occur between your general dentist and orthodontist. Night guards are usually fabricated at the general dentist's office, while retainers are part of the orthodontic treatment. A combination retainer/mouth guard can also be designed.

How long do I have to wear my retainer?

Regardless of whether orthodontic treatment happens in adolescence or adulthood, wearing a retainer indefinitely ensures the most stable result. After the initial period of nightly wear, retainer use can be cut back to two to three times a week. If treatment occurred decades ago and the bite remains stable, then once a week should be sufficient.

15

MUCH MORE THAN DRILL AND FILL

When a patient comes in for a routine checkup, one of the first questions the dentist asks is, "Are there any changes in your overall health?" The dentist also reviews the patient's current list of medications. The majority answer openly and willingly, but occasionally there's resistance. Some will invariably ask, "Why? What's that got to do with my teeth?"

As it turns out, the answer is, "A lot." Many medications reduce saliva flow and cause dry mouth, which increases the likelihood of cavities. A condition such as Parkinson's will lead to an eventual decline in the patient's ability to keep his mouth clean. Cancer treatments like targeted radiation and chemotherapy often result in a painful mouth and difficulty eating. Explaining these and other examples to patients helps them to understand the mouth-body connection.

Dentists are also in the perfect position to screen for other conditions. The average patient visits their dentist more regularly than any other health professional. So identifying a possible disease or other condition in the beginning stages often means earlier treatment and a more successful outcome.

SLEEP APNEA

Obstructive sleep apnea (OSA) occurs during sleep when insufficient air—and therefore oxygen—enters the body due to a constriction in the airway. Sometimes breathing stops entirely, followed by a gasp, after which breathing is resumed. Sleep is often marked by loud snoring. Sleep apnea sufferers wake up tired and may experience excessive daytime sleepiness. They may experience dry mouth from mouth breathing and snoring. Headaches are common due to the lack of oxygen.

The most obvious health ramification is waking up fatigued. This leads to a lack of focus, irritability, memory impairment, and an inability to concentrate on work or school. People with sleep apnea are 2.5 times more likely to be responsible for a motor vehicle accident.[1]

There are also less apparent health effects. Sleep apnea sufferers are at a higher risk of:

- Cardiovascular disease, including heart attack, stroke, and high blood pressure
- Diabetes
- Depression
- Dementia
- Obesity/weight gain

In general, the typical sleep apnea sufferer is an obese male with a large neck circumference and abdominal fat. That said, there are exceptions that include certain populations:

- Postmenopausal women (hormones may play a role)
- Children, although this is rare (discussed in chapter 12)
- Asians who don't fit the physical profile (It is thought that Asians may have craniofacial anatomic bony restrictions that limit the size of their airway.[2])

The Dentist's Role in Screening

Since sleep apnea stems from a narrow or reduced airway, the dentist is an appropriate health professional to evaluate this. Aside from basic knowledge, though, most dentists will need to seek additional training if they plan to treat patients in this area. This is no different from a dentist who wishes to place implants or provide Invisalign treatment. Although sleep medicine is not a recognized specialty, certain dentists choose to work primarily in this field. General screening can be done by any dentist, but should you require treatment for sleep apnea, ask your dentist for a referral to one of these practitioners.

The screening process begins with a simple question: Do you snore? Maybe it should be directed to the patient's bed partner, since that is the person who usually finds the snoring intolerable and insists on intervention. Not every snorer has sleep apnea, but the intensity of the snoring is correlated with the severity of the apnea.

The Physical Exam

The dentist will examine several locations:

- The soft palate/tonsillar area
- The size of the tongue in relation to the size of the mouth and its relative position in the mouth
- The mobility of the tongue and whether there's any tongue-tie
- The size of the jaws and any upper/lower jaw size discrepancy
- Any obstruction in the nostrils
- Any evidence of mouth breathing

The Questionnaire

The patient will be asked to answer a short questionnaire, such as the STOP-BANG or the Epworth Sleepiness Scale (ESS), where the results may indicate further testing. Common questions include:

- Have you ever fallen asleep while waiting at a traffic light?
- Has anyone observed you stop breathing during your sleep?
- Do you have or are you being treated for high blood pressure?

If your dentist suspects you may have sleep apnea, she will recommend further testing and refer you to a pulmonologist or sleep physician. The sleep study, or polysynography (PSG), is administered in one of two ways: a physician-supervised overnight study at a sleep lab or a home sleep test. The decision to do one over the other is now primarily an insurance-based financial one, but more detailed data is collected in the sleep lab study.

Treatment

Depending on the test results and severity of the obstructive sleep apnea (OSA), treatment may take one of several forms.

CPAP   Considered the gold standard of treatment, the CPAP (continuous positive airway pressure) machine is a device that fits over either the nose or the nose and mouth and delivers positive pressure oxygen. It's meant for moderate to severe cases. The CPAP needs to be individually fitted and monitored for effectiveness.

Mouth Guard   Ideal for mild to moderate cases of sleep apnea, a custom-made mouth guard (or mandibular advancement device) extends the lower jaw forward and opens the mouth. It, too, must be adjusted for proper fit and effectiveness. There is a risk that the bite will be irreversibly altered, and care must be taken to monitor this closely. A dentist with experience in sleep medicine should provide this treatment. Even though the care takes place in a dental setting, Medicare will often cover the expense for seniors.

Sleep Hygiene   Instituting good sleep habits forms the foundation for healthy sleep:

- Go to sleep and wake up at the same time each day.
- Avoid any electronics (TV, phone, etc.) in the bedroom.
- Sleep in a cool, darkened room.
- Avoid alcohol at least four hours prior to bedtime.
- Limit caffeine intake past lunchtime.
- If sleeping on your back triggers snoring, try sleeping on your side.
- Avoid daytime naps.

Cognitive Behavioral Therapy   Professional talk therapy may be needed to reinforce sleep hygiene habits or to manage nighttime awakenings and insomnia.

Accessory Devices Simple devices can sometimes make a difference. Over-the-counter nasal dilators expand the nostrils to allow for greater air intake. Taping over the lips keeps the mouth closed and may prevent or reduce mouth breathing and snoring. A small piece of tape placed vertically in the center of the mouth is preferable. Pillows or specially designed shirts aid with side sleeping. Over-the-counter tongue retaining or suctioning devices pull the tongue forward to open the airway and possibly reduce snoring. In general, they are not that well tolerated.

Surgery Anatomic causes of sleep apnea may be surgically corrected. For example, extremely large tonsils and adenoids that block the airway can be removed, or a deviated septum that prevents adequate nasal breathing can be straightened.

ORAL CANCER

Every year about fifty-four thousand cases of oral or oropharyngeal cancer are diagnosed in the United States, and there are more than eleven thousand annual deaths from this type of cancer.[3] It is most frequently found in the tongue, the tonsils and oropharynx, the gums, and the floor of the mouth. Common types of oral and oropharyngeal cancers include squamous cell carcinoma—the predominant one—salivary gland tumors, and lymphomas.

There are several specific risk factors associated with oral cancer:

- *Smoking and drinking:* We all know that smoking—cigarettes, cigars, pipes, snuff, betel nut, and other tobacco products—increases the risk of cancer in many parts of the body. The role of alcohol is less well understood but the link between heavy alcohol consumption and oral, oropharyngeal, esophageal, and liver cancer is well established. Smoking and alcohol use together multiply the risk of oral cancer. One study showed that people who drank heavily and smoked had a three hundred–times higher risk of upper aerodigestive tract—including lips, mouth, tongue, and throat—cancers than people who did neither.[4]
- *Human papillomavirus:* HPV is actually a whole family of viruses that are transmitted sexually. HPV cancers are often found in the

back of the tongue, tonsils, and oropharyngeal areas. As such, they're more difficult to detect.

- *Gender:* Oral cancers are more commonly found in men.
- *Age:* With the exception of HPV-related cancers, these malignancies occur more commonly in people over age fifty-five. HPV cancers, however, can afflict younger patients.
- *Sunlight exposure:* People exposed to significant UV radiation are at higher risk of cancer in the lip area.

The Dentist's Role in Screening

An oral cancer screening should be performed by your dentist every time you have a cleaning and examination. If this doesn't happen, find a new dentist. The screening should include:

- A visual examination of the soft tissues in your mouth, including the oropharyngeal area
- A manual palpation to feel for any swelling
- Checking the lymph nodes in the neck for any enlargement
- A tongue examination with your tongue sticking out
- X-ray analysis

You will probably be referred to an oral surgeon if the screening unearths anything suspicious. A biopsy may be performed and the sample sent to an oral pathologist for diagnosis. Additional X-rays may also be taken.

A diagnosis of cancer may involve several treatment pathways. It might be a simple procedure such as removal of a small lesion. More often, treatment may include radiation, chemotherapy, or surgery, and each affects the mouth in specific ways.

Surgery   When major surgery leaves the patient with a sizeable defect, an artificial prosthesis like a denture can be made. But in the past, these wouldn't always stay in place and suffered from the same problems as all dentures, only more so. Now, implants can be used to attach the prosthesis to bone, making the appliance more stable and functional. Sophisticated scanners and 3D printers can even create custom pieces of jawbone from titanium.

Radiation   Radiation in the head and neck area must be preceded by a thorough dental exam. A decision needs to be made about any compromised teeth—and that is usually to take them out. Extraction after radiation harbors substantial risk for osteoradionecrosis, a spontaneous process that results in infection and the uncontrolled loss of healthy jawbone.

If the salivary glands are in the field of radiation, indefinite reduced saliva flow may result. Mouth sores may develop, making eating painful and difficult. The mouth rinses described in chapter 6 can alleviate some of the symptoms.

Chemotherapy   Depending on the specific chemotherapy regimen, dry mouth and mouth sores may also be a problem. Additionally, there may be changes in taste that linger beyond the time of treatment. Historically, long-term chemotherapy has limited effectiveness with squamous cell carcinoma, the most common form of oral cancer. Research in immunology and pharmacology shows promise with newer biologic therapies.

GRINDING AND CLENCHING

Both grinding and clenching fall under the category of parafunctional behavior, where the normal function is chewing. But there's a difference between the two. Grinding, or bruxism, is the habitual, often unintentional, rubbing back and forth of upper and lower teeth. Not only is this behavior very loud—it can sometimes even be heard from another room or even another floor—but over time it results in the wearing down of the teeth. As the outer layer of enamel thins or disappears, the teeth can become sensitive to cold liquids and foods, and even to cold air. Clenching, by contrast, is the silent, forceful gritting together of upper and lower teeth. It is also habitual and often unintentional. Clenchers tend to break teeth rather than wear them down. Specifically, the lower second molars and upper premolars are most likely to fracture, sometimes into two hopeless segments where the only option is extraction.

The causes of grinding or clenching are not fully understood. It's often linked to stress and anxiety. Certain medications, including antidepressants known as SSRIs (selective serotonin reuptake inhibitors), result in grinding, as do drugs like cocaine and ecstasy. Bruxism is also related to sleep apnea.

Grinding is often overdiagnosed. Over the years I've heard this repeatedly: "My previous dentist told me I grind my teeth and I need a mouth guard." When I peer into their mouths, more often than not, I see little evidence of grinding. Tooth wear is not synonymous with grinding. It can also be the result of:

- Acid reflux, also known as GERD (gastroesophageal reflux disease)
- Frequent eating of highly acidic foods, such as lemons or grapefruits
- Drinking acidic carbonated beverages

Wear on specific teeth can be the aftermath of an oral habit like nail biting or pencil chewing, or unusual wear could have occurred prior to orthodontic treatment, when the teeth were misaligned.

The tooth wear from clenching differs significantly from that of bruxing. With clenching, the lower second molars typically exhibit a dished-out appearance, where the chewing surface is shaped like a shallow bowl. The tongue may have reverse scallops along its outer edge that correspond to the rounded curves of the teeth. Grinding results in the uniform wearing away of all the teeth, sometimes to the point where they are flattened.

To help determine whether you grind or clench, ask yourself these questions:

- Do you clench or grind exclusively during the day?
- Do you grind or clench your teeth while sleeping?

You may say, "I'm sleeping. How do I know?" Indications may include waking up with a sore jaw, ear or TMJ pain, an inability to open your mouth fully, or diffuse and generalized pain in the teeth that's unrelated to a cavity or any identifiable source. There are apps available that will record any sounds made during sleep. While this can be useful in the diagnosis of grinding, remember that clenching is silent. You can also consider videoing yourself during sleep. The camera should be focused tightly on your face since clenching will be evident with the contraction of the masseter and temporalis muscles. Alternatively, ask someone to watch as you're sleeping.

Treatment

Daytime Grinders and Clenchers Now that you've been made aware of this unconscious behavior, the first step in treating daytime clenching or grinding is to notice every time you're doing it. Try to keep a log. Under what circumstances and how frequently does it happen? If there's a pattern, perhaps you can make a change to avoid putting yourself in that situation. For example, if a friend always sets your teeth on edge, try to limit your contact with that person.

Behavior modification is key. As with any new behavior, being aware is the first step to transform it into habit.

- Open your mouth slightly so your jaw is relaxed and your teeth are apart in a resting position. Unless you are eating, your upper and lower teeth should never be touching.
- Place the tip of your tongue on the roof of your mouth, behind but not touching the upper front teeth. That is the ideal home position for the tongue. With the tongue there, it's almost impossible to grind or clench your teeth.

You don't need a mouth guard. It's highly impractical to wear one consistently during waking hours unless you have a job that requires little to no verbal interaction.

Nighttime Grinders and Clenchers Because nighttime grinding and clenching happens while you are asleep, a mouth guard (occlusal splint) is critical to treating it. But not just any mouth guard will do.

- You need a custom-made hard acrylic mouth guard. Avoid the over-the-counter, do-it-yourself products. Don't use your bleaching tray or Invisalign tray as a mouth guard, as they are neither thick nor protective. If you're currently wearing an orthodontic retainer, a combination retainer/mouth guard can be easily made.

- It must be fitted and adjusted as needed for comfort. The bite must be even, and adjusted as necessary, with the mouth guard in place.
- Periodically, the mouth guard should be checked to ensure the fit and bite are stable.
- Some nighttime bruxism is related to sleep apnea. Consider getting screened and tested.

What if your teeth show typical signs of wear but you don't know if you grind or clench? Perhaps the wear is the result of a previous stressful period and you think you no longer grind your teeth. Have a mouth guard made anyway. After a few weeks, there will be evidence on the appliance itself if you're grinding or clenching. Besides, if you're prone to bruxism during stressful periods, the mouth guard won't go to waste, as stress will likely assert itself again.

If you need future dental work—say, a crown—the mouth guard can almost always be retrofitted to accommodate the new restoration. This applies to mouth guards for sleep apnea as well.

TEMPOROMANDIBULAR JOINT DISORDERS

The mandible has two temporomandibular joints, a right and a left one. Temporomandibular joint disorders (TMD) affect the function of one or both joints and are almost always accompanied by pain and tenderness in the surrounding region. TMDs are also marked by an inability to open the mouth to its full extent. This group of disorders is mistakenly referred to by the public as TMJ; however, TMJ stands for the joint itself. Although TMDs have a host of causes, perhaps the most interesting is that it's often a mystery. TMDs can occur in a number of circumstances:

- *Arthritis in the joint:* Arthritis can occur in any joint in the body, including the TMJ. This often has a hereditary component.
- *Trauma:* Injury to one or both joints can occur with a fall, a car accident, or a physical altercation. The symptoms often—but not always—appear shortly after the traumatic incident. As un-

traumatic as it seemingly appears, trauma can even occur from sleeping in an uncomfortable position. As a result of a poor night's sleep, I experienced pain and tenderness in one of my TMJs once. After a few days to a week, the discomfort gradually subsided and then resolved.

- *Deterioration or damage in the joint or joint capsule:* There is a disc behind the joint that sometimes gets displaced or torn. A crackling, grating sensation or sound called crepitus may indicate damage in the joint or surrounding disc and cartilage.
- *Damage to surrounding muscles, ligaments, or neighboring anatomy:* Spasms in the masseter, the largest chewing muscle in the face, can cause TMJ pain. Because the ear is directly behind the TMJ, an ear infection can also cause pain in the TMJ area.
- *Bruxism:* Teeth grinding can lead to TMD, as can clenching.
- *Headaches:* Headaches or migraines can be associated with TMD. The relationship between headaches, migraines, and TMD is not well understood.
- *Other physical ailments:* Conditions such as sleep apnea (where teeth grinding can occur), back pain, fibromyalgia, and irritable bowel syndrome are all associated with TMD.
- *Unknown causes:* With TMD, it's not unusual that a cause can't be identified.

Because the causes are varied and hard to pinpoint, stick to the most conservative plan. Unless you're in excruciating pain, initially it is best to do nothing except for what's recommended in the "Non-invasive Recommendations" section below. Most TMD symptoms resolve spontaneously over time. While you're "doing nothing," spend your time researching a qualified TMD specialist with a proven track record of success in case your symptoms persist. Clicking and popping noises don't require examination or treatment unless they are accompanied by pain.

Many dentists will automatically offer a mouth guard as the treatment of choice. The truth is that most dentists, myself included, either aren't trained in this area or were trained with information that is now outdated. The other truth is that you'll probably get better with or without the mouth guard.

Noninvasive Recommendations

Conservative measures can be taken to reduce TMJ pain:

- Stick to soft foods.
- Avoid foods that force you to open your mouth too wide, like three-inch deli sandwiches.
- Don't chew gum for hours on end.
- Use warm, moist compresses in the joint area.
- Take nonsteroidal anti-inflammatories, such as ibuprofen, as needed. Be aware that anti-inflammatory medications may upset your stomach.

Treatment

Diagnosis must be determined prior to treatment. However, broadly recognized and standardized criteria for diagnosis don't really exist. Unlike a pregnancy test, there's no one test to determine whether you have TMD. Information gathering should include a physical examination of the affected and surrounding areas, an evaluation of the patient's symptoms, and X-rays or imaging such as an MRI or CT scan.

Treatment is dependent on the cause of the TMD, if it can be clearly identified. Aside from the noninvasive options, several treatment options are available:

- *Physical therapy:* Physical therapy may increase the jaw's range of motion and improve surrounding muscle function.
- *Relaxation methods:* Stress and anxiety sometimes contribute to habits that can cause TMJ pain and dysfunction. Relaxation methods that may help include exercise, yoga, cognitive behavioral therapy, antianxiety medications or muscle relaxants, and relaxation and meditation techniques. Usually this treatment involves a combination of strategies.
- *Mouth guard or occlusal splint:* An occlusal splint serves multiple purposes. It relaxes the facial muscles, takes the pressure off the joints themselves, and eliminates any muscle spasms that contribute to symptoms. In essence, the splint serves to deprogram the area, allowing for a more symptom-free baseline to deter-

mine next steps. All dentists make mouth guards, but you should seek out a dentist who has experience treating TMD.

- *Surgery:* Surgery should be a last resort. Proceed cautiously with any irreversible surgical procedure, whether it's arthroscopic or invasive. When I was a dental student, I watched many TMJ surgeries where the joint was cut off and removed. To my knowledge, this proved to be an ineffective long-term solution. Today, in cases of advanced joint damage, a sectioned TMJ can be replaced with an implant. Discuss any surgical options with your TMD specialist and surgeon.
- *Botox:* Although the injection of Botox is currently not an FDA-approved TMD treatment, it has been used to reduce muscle spasms around the TMJ. A review of the studies done shows Botox has some therapeutic benefit, although more rigorous research is needed.[5]

MORE MOUTH-BODY CONNECTIONS

Your dentist may be the first to notice other emerging health conditions. If he brings it up, resist the urge to say, "How do you know? You're not a 'real' doctor." While it's accurate that your dentist doesn't possess a medical degree, he nevertheless has undergone some level of medical training. He's not providing a final diagnosis, but merely alerting you to follow up with your physician. In fact, he's doing you a favor and looking out for your overall health.

Diabetes

The relationship between gum disease and diabetes is reciprocal. Diabetics are more likely to have uncontrolled gum disease and gum disease makes sugar control more difficult. If a patient's gum disease worsens suddenly, type 2 diabetes may play a role.

Dementia

A longtime patient calls for directions to the office. In a matter of minutes, she calls again. There may be a half dozen phone calls in which she asks the same thing. This scenario, which happened more than once in my practice, is a surefire hint of impending cognitive decline. Another is the patient who always brings a notebook and writes down everything the dentist says. He may downplay this, saying something like, "I just want to get the facts straight" or "I want to be able to review this later." In my experience, patients can expertly hide their cognitive deterioration from family members for a long time. Sometimes intervention is required to ensure their safety.

High Blood Pressure

Many dental offices will take blood pressure on a new patient or during a checkup. Since there are rarely symptoms with high blood pressure, this is a quick and easy screening that alerts the patient to seek further medical attention.

Anemia

A hallmark of anemia is very pale gums, as opposed to the normal reddish color. If the patient also confirms she's been extremely tired lately, a visit to her physician may be indicated.

Gastric Reflux (GERD)

Exposure to stomach acid, which happens with chronic gastric reflux, will damage the teeth in a specific pattern. An astute dentist can spot this right away.

Headaches, Migraines, and Trigeminal Neuralgia

Headache, migraine, and trigeminal neuralgia are all conditions associated with varying degrees of pain. (Botox has provided relief for each of these.) Trigeminal neuralgia is a rare ailment marked by unpredictable episodes of excruciating pain, sometimes brought on by nothing more than a slight breeze to the face. In general, pain signals are complex and subjective. Pain can also be referred from the point of origin to another location, making diagnosis challenging. Once it's determined that pain is not coming from a tooth or elsewhere in your mouth, then a nondental source must be considered. Your dentist may refer you to either an orofacial pain specialist or your physician.

Sexually Transmitted Diseases

Besides HPV, gonorrhea, herpes, chlamydia, and syphilis can exhibit mouth or lip sores. Some of these diseases are curable; all of them should be treated and managed.

COVID-19

In the mouth, COVID-19 may present with a loss of taste; mouth sores; or, more rarely, osteonecrosis, the spontaneous sloughing of healthy jawbone. Chances are, you'll have other symptoms that point to COVID, but if your dentist notices any of these signs, you should follow up with your physician.

WHAT ELSE CAN YOUR DENTIST DETECT?

In addition to disease states, there are certain instances where behavior or the body itself displays hints that all is not well with a patient. Again, because of the close physical proximity, dentists are in the perfect position to identify situations that may be harmful to patients. They can speak directly to the patient or alert the appropriate parties.

Eating Disorders

In bulimics, the backs of the upper and lower front teeth tend to erode as a result of sustained exposure to vomit. The skilled dentist is a diplomat and a detective in differentiating between acid reflux and bulimia.

Mental Health Issues

I have always felt that my job is part dentist and part therapist. Due to the intimate nature of the relationship, many patients experience a special bond and trust with their dentist. Patients have shared with me private information about their spouses, children, or extended family. Occasionally they talked about their mental health. A caring and astute dentist should recognize when their patients are vulnerable and possibly suggest follow-up with a medical professional.

Drug Use

Suspected drug use is another diplomatic minefield, but again, a caring dentist is acting in the patient's best interest by bringing this subject up. Patients addicted to opioids will use every excuse to seek a prescription. "Meth mouth" is a documented consequence of methamphetamine addiction characterized by rampant tooth decay. Likewise, daily marijuana users may develop cavities from frequent snacking. A listless person showing no affect may be addicted to more serious drugs.

Child, Elder, and Domestic Abuse

Over the years, more than one senior citizen has handed over her checkbook to my front office manager with instructions to "fill in the blanks, dear." We marveled that they were so trusting—and how easily they could be taken advantage of. These vulnerable populations can't protect themselves.

The legal requirements for dentists to report suspected abuse vary from state to state, but many states require all licensed healthcare providers—including dentists—to report domestic violence, physical assault, suspected child abuse or neglect, and suspected elder abuse or neglect. Regardless of the law, dentists have an ethical obligation to follow up in these situations.

Human Trafficking

In the United States, human trafficking is estimated to be a $150 billion a year business.[6] Remember when missing children were featured on milk cartons? Due to the hidden nature of this crime, reliable statistics are hard to determine, but it's thought that at any given time, 4.8 million people worldwide are commercially forced into sexual labor.[7] Many of these are children who must be kept in a relatively healthy condition. It behooves the criminals to have a tooth infection treated. Dentists are in a perfect position to spot a child who never makes eye contact, an accompanying adult who isn't related, or a child who appears fearful of the accompanying adult. Again, this is another vulnerable group where an observant and caring dentist can change a life.

Dentistry is about so much more than drill and fill. With their medical training, dentists are the ideal healthcare professionals to check for conditions which affect the rest of the body. And a healthy mouth is about so much more than healthy teeth. It encompasses the entire oral cavity—teeth, gums, tongue, bones, joints, sinuses, throat, and soft tissues—a part of the body that communicates with the rest of the person. Information, nutrition, and microorganisms are constantly exchanged, and warnings routinely appear in the mouth of any developing diseases. Your dentist does—and should—play an important role in the management of your overall health and well-being.

16

WILL YOUR FUTURE DENTIST
BE A ROBOT?

It may be shocking to hear, but when I first began working, dentists didn't wear gloves. This changed with the advent of the AIDS epidemic, when infection control became a serious matter overnight. Instruments were either sterilized or single use. Surfaces were disinfected. What couldn't be adequately sanitized was covered in a plastic wrap–like material. The recent COVID-19 pandemic added more protections for patient and dentist alike: air purification devices, plexiglass barriers, and N95 masks.

In the past few decades, dentistry has experienced many changes and advances. Some of the more notable advances have been discussed in previous chapters. These include:

- The popularity of implants to replace missing teeth
- New and improved materials allowing for tooth-colored fillings and aesthetic crowns
- Digital radiography, allowing X-rays that can be taken more quickly and with less radiation
- CAD/CAM dentistry, allowing a crown to be started and completed in one appointment
- Aligner orthodontics

- Awareness of the mouth-body connection with conditions such as heart disease, sleep apnea, and diabetes
- The pervasive influence of the internet, enabling dentists to use websites and social media

Going forward, progress will take place on many fronts. Specifically, artificial intelligence (AI) and digital dentistry will play a role. Greater understanding of our individual genetic makeup and biology will lead to pharmacological and immunological advances. These disciplines dovetail together; for example, by using currently available scans, images, and biomarkers, we may be able to predict the future growth of a tumor.

ARTIFICIAL INTELLIGENCE

First used in 1950, the term "artificial intelligence" simply means machines that are able to mimic human functions and behavior. The field of AI is constantly evolving. In machine learning (ML), a category of AI, algorithms are generated to discern patterns from vast quantities of data and used to perform tasks. Sometimes the algorithms are static; other times they change as a response to the data.

AI affects every aspect of our lives, from the advertising that pops up on our laptops to the facial recognition that identifies us at the US Customs kiosk at the airport. Often we're not even aware of AI's ubiquity and impact.

In October 2020, a fifteen-member Dental AI Council was formed by dental leaders and innovators. According to its website, the council's mission is to "advance research, education and thought leadership that helps answer those questions, while bringing clarity and foresight to the discourse surrounding AI's role in the dental industry of tomorrow."[1]

Challenges of AI

In what was once depicted only in science fiction movies, AI is becoming increasingly commonplace. Yet the field is not without its challenges, many of which are significant and must be overcome.

Data Security and Transparency Due to its sensitive nature, medical data should be confidential and anonymous. But in order for AI to be effective, data must be shared widely across different fields, institutions, and even countries. Data breaches are a reality and skepticism that medical data can indeed be kept private remains an issue. The flip side is the lack of transparency with anonymous data. AI is all about good data, but without transparency, it's difficult to determine the quality and completeness of the data from which ML algorithms are generated. Since predictions and decisions are based upon these algorithms, how can we be sure that the data are sound?

Data Biases AI is used to diagnose disease, recommend treatment, and predict outcomes. It's tempting for doctors to take this information at face value without questioning the basis of this "thinking." In 2019 the FDA formulated an action plan to treat AI and ML software as a medical device.[2] For practitioners, such "medical devices" should never be relied upon exclusively, but instead used in conjunction with their knowledge, experience, and clinical skills.

Cost Creating new technology is a significant investment in terms of cost, time, and human resources. Obtaining and implementing new technology is equally expensive, particularly for small business owners such as dentists. With rapidly changing technology, resources must also be devoted to ongoing training, critical evaluation of the products, and maintenance.

DIGITAL DENTISTRY

Digital dentistry is the process of using computer-controlled equipment to perform dental procedures that were once done mechanically or manually. Successful digital dentistry processes have been incorporated into practice and become mainstream. One example is digital radiography, which has replaced darkroom development of X-rays. Now, using a computer and software, a tooth is scanned and an image appears almost instantaneously on the screen.

Other mainstream digital dentistry processes include CAD/CAM crowns, digital impression taking, and intraoral cameras. This area is constantly changing with the introduction of new processes and products.

Before incorporating new digital technology into their practice, dentists must evaluate whether the new technology truly improves patient care, factoring in the cost and time involved. Take the intraoral camera, for instance. There's a reason they say, "A picture is worth a thousand words." With one photograph, a dentist can show and explain to her patient what's going on with a particular tooth. This facilitates better communication, increased clarity, and may motivate the patient to commit to treatment. It is no wonder that almost all dentists now use intraoral cameras.

Similar to AI technology, the cost of acquiring, training, and implementation represents a challenge. Investment in new equipment generally comes out of the practice profits. Purchasing a $1,000 intraoral camera is markedly different from buying or leasing a $50,000 CAD/CAM machine or a $500,000 3D printer. In addition, the time and costs to implement new systems and provide training tax an already busy staff.

PHARMACOLOGY, IMMUNOLOGY, AND YOU

Cancer treatment has traditionally involved some combination of surgery, chemotherapy, and radiation therapy. While the same modalities still exist, today the body's genetic code and immune system can be used to create specific chemotherapeutic agents. No longer will medications be a one-size-fits-all approach.

The Cancer Genome Atlas program has discovered molecular signaling pathways—instructions within the cell—in squamous cell oral cancers. So far, ongoing research has identified drugs that inhibit signals within these pathways to shrink tumors. Likewise, edits to our genetic code can alter the way our bodies respond to cancer caused by HPV.

Our immune systems can also be used to tailor medication. Chemotherapeutic agents can directly target immune cells—the ones which fight bacteria, viruses, and other invaders—to inhibit tumor growth.

In diagnosis, biomarkers found in our saliva can be used to perform a biopsy. Instead of a traditional surgical biopsy which may cause inflammation, you might get a "liquid" biopsy where a disease will be diagnosed from your saliva.

Much of this area is being studied and under research, but the intersection of pharmacology and immunology holds great promise and opportunity for customized disease treatment.

NEW DENTAL APPLICATIONS

You may be wondering exactly what AI or immunology has to do with going to the dentist. There are countless ways these technologies can be used in dentistry, limited only by our imagination. Although some are still in the research phase, the potential is truly exciting.

Diagnosis

Dentists need to process a lot of information in a relatively short time. In an exam, he must evaluate each tooth individually and as part of the entire mouth, the gums and other soft tissue, the jaws, and X-rays—and talk to the patient about any symptoms or concerning issues (and catch up on her family news since the last visit). Under these conditions it is understandable that a hard-to-see cavity might be missed. AI technology is perfect for reviewing vast quantities of information quickly and precisely.

- AI has been shown to be adept at diagnosing cavities, even surpassing human accuracy.[3] Combine that with its speed, and what dentist wouldn't want to use it?
- In root canals, critical anatomic measurements are achievable through AI. The more accurate the measurements, the greater the prognosis for saving the tooth.
- AI is especially good at identifying teeth and can easily identify extra teeth.
- AI can also detect early osteoporosis in the jaw and osteoarthritis in the temporomandibular joint.[4]
- AI algorithms have shown promise in the early detection of head and neck cancers. Early diagnosis makes possible early treatment

and more positive outcomes. Using saliva and ML, the Viome saliva test can screen for squamous cell carcinoma in the mouth and oropharyngeal area, the most common oral cancer.[5] In 2021 Viome received FDA Breakthrough Device Designation for this new technology.

- AI can also classify cell types and differentiate tumor grades.

Predictive Diagnosis

While the idea of discovering whether we might develop oral cancer in the future may be appealing, remember that AI is all about good data. The assumption is that the data are accurate and relevant to the questions being asked. Until the field of AI can reconcile the need for medical data privacy with the need for data transparency, the area of predictive diagnosis remains a work in progress.

Dentists should also incorporate this information as one element in their treatment decisions rather than relying solely on AI predictions.

- Using a patient's scans and images, AI can predict the growth and size of a tumor. While this application is still in the research phase, this information may be used to decide on the aggressiveness of the treatment.
- AI can use data to predict the likelihood of oral cancers or pre-cancers in currently disease-free individuals. With this knowledge, higher-risk patients may want to get examined more frequently.
- Algorithms can predict the sizes of unerupted teeth,[6] which may be useful in planning orthodontic treatment.
- ML algorithms that incorporate socioeconomic factors such as age and income can be used to predict future tooth loss.

Clinical Treatment

The practice of dentistry has changed dramatically in the last thirty years. Where dental students were once taught how to make crowns with the lost-wax process, now they are creating crowns with a keyboard and CAD/CAM machine. There will be even more changes ahead, both in terms of digital dentistry and improved materials.

- When an impression is needed, instead of the "goop" you've been accustomed to, a scanner can take images and translate them into a three-dimensional replica of your mouth.
- When selecting a color for a crown, almost every dentist finds it challenging to exactly match the patient's other teeth. AI can easily accomplish this task.
- Rather than using an educated guess for implant placement, computed-assisted technology can now help your surgeon identify the ideal implant location. It can even determine multiple implant placement sites that work together for a multi-implant attached denture. In the future, a real-time navigation system may be used for implant placement.
- Although it is not commonly done currently, the technology exists for 3D printing of dental appliances such as mouth guards and dentures. Recently, a custom titanium jaw was created for a cancer surgery patient using 3D printing that matched the original bone's size and weight.[7] The new jaw was anchored onto the remaining existing jaw with implants.
- In orthodontic treatment, digital dentistry and AI are used to plan the treatment and create the series of trays and attachments for aligner orthodontics. With metal braces, custom brackets can be designed and 3D printed.
- In the field of immunotherapeutics, new drugs such as pembrolizumab and nivolumab have been shown to slow tumor growth.[8] Squamous cell oral cancers eventually resist currently available chemotherapy medications, so the developments in this area are welcome and promising.
- Gene-editing technology such as clustered regularly interspaced short palindromic repeats (CRISPRs) has been used to target specific gene regions in the treatment of HPV cancers. They either reduce the virus responsible for HPV cancers or make them more amenable to treatment by the newer pharmacological immunotherapies.[9]

Smart Products

Toothbrushes Employing a downloadable app and AI, smart toothbrushes can provide input on your brushing technique and habits. They can detect pressure, motion, and surfaces covered and can even adjust automatically if you're brushing too hard. They can track your total brushing time and brushing history, to be reviewed later with your dentist or hygienist. Some smart brushes can record your brushing and provide coaching tips or praise.

Since these brushes can run into the hundreds of dollars, it may be a worthwhile purchase only if you'll actually use all the features.

Bad Breath Detection Researchers have developed a small, thumb-sized prototype to detect bad breath (halitosis) in real time.[10] Using nanofibers, the device measures hydrogen sulfide in exhaled breath. Larger devices also exist to measure bad breath, some more reliably than others.

Delivery and Management of Care

Teledentistry The technology for remote medical appointments has been around for years, but the COVID-19 pandemic accelerated telemedicine's popularity and use. Obviously much of dentistry must be performed inperson. However, information gathering and some preliminary diagnosis can be done through teledentistry. Likewise, consultations and a discussion of examination findings can be conducted remotely.

Electronic Dental Records Dentists have been slow to change to electronic health records, in part because the government financial incentives largely did not apply to them. When electronic health records were introduced, the hope was that healthcare providers and hospitals would be able to access the same patient records seamlessly. In reality, however, only individual hospital groups and their affiliated physician members have access, whereas a different hospital group may not. Dentists are also outside this loop.

One potential advantage of electronic records is that reliable anonymized data might be available for AI databases. Patient privacy is rightly a concern that curtails this access to data. Furthermore, the anonymity of the data makes it hard to determine its reliability.

Digital Communication from Your Dentist Just as you might get reminders from OpenTable regarding a dinner reservation, you may be receiving text messages or emails from your dentist on a regular basis to remind you of upcoming appointments and communicate other information. Many patients find this a more convenient way to communicate with their dentist and other healthcare providers.

Insurance Processing Insurance claims are now processed electronically for faster turnaround and payment. Insurance companies also use AI to approve treatment in realtime and to audit for insurance fraud.

Appointment Scheduling and Remote Bill Paying You may have the option to remotely schedule appointments and pay bills—and more—if your dentist has a system that enables an online account.

CURRENTLY IN RESEARCH

It's tempting to read a headline that may say "Now You Can Grow Teeth" and conclude that your broken tooth will repair itself. While it's true that enamel may be produced in a laboratory environment, it's an undifferentiated blob, and the technology has not been perfected much less completely researched. Keep this in mind as headlines tout breakthroughs.

New Dental Pulp

Every year 15 million root canals are done in the United States. While this procedure saves the tooth, removal of the dental pulp, consisting of nerves, blood cells, and fibrous tissue, makes the tooth more brittle and prone to breakage. Researchers have developed a hydrogel that works with a person's stem cells to re-create the dental pulp.[11] It is injected directly into the root canal space. This product is currently in animal trials.

Growing Enamel

When you break an arm, the bone repairs itself. When you cut your finger accidentally, the skin heals. Enamel, the hardest substance in the human body, doesn't have the same capability. When a tooth gets a cavity, the outer layer of enamel cannot repair itself.

Scientists have long struggled with creating artificial enamel, which consists of a complex geometric matrix of ingredients. But recently researchers designed an artificial enamel that is stronger than the real thing.[12] It's not quite ready for practical use, though. The material must be heated to 300°C, then frozen and carefully cut with a diamond saw. As promising as this substance is to repair teeth, your average dental office isn't equipped to handle the significant processing requirements. (Artificial enamel could be used outside the mouth, for example, to protect cell phones when accidentally dropped.)

Meanwhile, researchers at the University of Washington have developed a lozenge of genetically engineered enamel building blocks. Each lozenge deposits several microns (one human hair is approximately 70 microns) that can bind to damaged enamel.[13] The therapeutic applications of this product remain to be seen.

Dental Robots

Robin is a cute robot who puts children at ease by playing games and singing songs. Robin also educates in a kid-friendly way with animations.[14] YOMI, the first FDA-approved computerized navigation robotic system, was created to assist surgeons with placing implants more accurately.[15]

Robots are ideal for handling repetitive, labor-intensive tasks consistently. In dentistry, many such tasks exist. For example, despite its tediousness, the cleaning and sterilization of instruments must be done with care every single time. A robot may even be superior to a dental assistant, who might perform this task hurriedly at the end of a long workday.

While Robin and YOMI currently exist, areas where robots may play a future role include:

- Robot-assisted cancer surgery, particularly in difficult-to-access spaces like the back of the mouth, throat, and base of the tongue
- Robot-assisted surgery for sleep apnea to correct anatomic obstructions
- The manufacture of dentures or partial dentures, including the placement and waxing of artificial teeth
- The bending of orthodontic wire for maximum effect
- In lieu of a human dental assistant, taking X-rays and scans by placing the X-rays directly into patients' mouths
- Training dental students in patient simulations
- Testing of dental materials for durability and wear with a dental simulator

However exciting the possibilities are, the challenges are nevertheless significant. First, the development and implementation of any robotic system is very expensive. Robots also require skill to operate and maintain. The information that forms the foundational "brain" of the robot is critical, particularly if the robot is tasked with making any clinical decisions. And in addition to the robotic system itself, there are the real-world uncertainties of whether patients or dentists will accept a robot's treatment or contribution. Many people would rather speak to a live person than a computer. Finally, much more research needs to be conducted in this area.

Some of the practices described in this chapter are commonplace and accepted. Others are still in the research phase. Still others are merely ideas at the moment. One thing is certain: Technological change will occur. My hope is that it will happen in a positive, productive, and healthy way.

ACKNOWLEDGMENTS

I've always wanted to be a writer but didn't know how to start, or if I could even string more than two words together. Thank you to Paddy Calistro and Scott McAuley for providing early guidance. And I couldn't have launched this project without Leslie Lehr, who showed me the nuts and bolts of how to become a published author.

Thank you to my agent, Nancy Rosenfeld, for finding a home for this book. To Suzanne Staszak-Silva, Anne Cushman, Joanna Wattenberg, Veronica Dove, and everyone at Rowman & Littlefield, I'm grateful for your expertise. To Meghann French, thank you for turning my manuscript into a book.

To respected orthodontist Dr. Jeff Jang, thank you for reviewing the chapter on orthodontics.

Thanks to my husband John for supporting me, figuratively and literally, through this endeavor. And to my children, Danielle (and Bryan) and Spencer (and Lucia), who both work in tech and not in dentistry. Thanks for the technical support.

And finally, thank you to all the patients whom it's been my privilege and honor to treat. You're the best!

CHAPTER 6

1. Yogita Datta, "The U.S. Toothpaste Market: A Competitive Profile," *Journal of Economics and Public Finance* 6, no. 1 (February 27, 2020): 1, https://www.researchgate.net/publication/339538350_The_US_Toothpaste _Market_A_Competitive_Profile.

2. Datta, "The U.S. Toothpaste Market," 10.

3. Robert H. Smerling, "Tossing Flossing?" *Harvard Health Blog*, August 17, 2016, https://www.health.harvard.edu/blog/tossing-floss ing-2016081710196.

4. Catherine Saint Louis, "Feeling Guilty about Not Flossing? Maybe There's No Need," *New York Times*, August 2, 2016, https://www.nytimes .com/2016/08/03/health/flossing-teeth-cavities.html.

5. Sanjay Gupta, *Keep Sharp: Build a Better Brain at Any Age* (New York: Simon & Schuster, 2021).

6. American Academy of Periodontology, "New Study Suggests the Ideal Sequence for Removing Plaque," press release, August 29, 2018, https:// www.perio.org/press-release/new-study-suggests-the-ideal-sequence-for -removing-plaque/.

7. Vagish Kumar L. Shanbhag, "Oil Pulling for Maintaining Oral Hygiene—A Review," *Journal of Traditional and Complementary Medicine* 7, no. 1 (January 2017): 106–109, https://www.ncbi.nlm.nih.gov/pmc/articles /PMC5198813/.

CHAPTER 7

1. EINPresswire, "Cosmetic Dentistry Market Size to Worth USD 35.66 Billion in 2028," press release, June 22, 2022, https://www.einnews.com/pr _news/577915674/cosmetic-dentistry-market-size-to-worth-usd-35-66 -billion-in-2028-at-a-cagr-of-6-3-says-reports-and-data.

2. What's Cooking America, "Teeth Whitening," accessed June 22, 2022, https://whatscookingamerica.net/healthbeauty/teethwhit ening.htm#:~:text=According%20to%20the%20American%20 Academy,whitening%20products%20last%20year%20alone.

3. Leandro Feliz-Matos, Luis Miguel Hernandez, and Ninoska Abreu, "Dental Bleaching Techniques; Hydrogen-Carbamide Peroxides and Light Sources for Activation, an Update," *Open Dentistry Journal* 8 (2014): 264–68, https:// www.ncbi.nlm.nih.gov/pmc/articles/PMC4311381/.

4. Arti S. Naidu et al., "Over-the-Counter Tooth Whitening Agents: A Review of Literature," *Brazilian Dental Journal* 31, no. 3 (May–June 2020), https://www.scielo.br/j/bdj/a/yjx5CcCCQzRWqhzFKVSgVVK/?lang=en.

CHAPTER 8

1. Yogita Datta, "The U.S. Toothpaste Market: A Competitive Profile," *Journal of Economics and Public Finance* 6, no. 1 (February 27, 2020): 150, https://www.researchgate.net/publication/339538350_The_US_Toothpaste_Market_A_Competitive_Profile.

2. Fiona MacDonald, "Evidence Is Mounting That Routine Wisdom Teeth Removal Is a Waste of Time," *Science Alert*, October 28, 2016, https://www.sciencealert.com/no-you-probably-don-t-need-to-get-your-wisdom-teeth-removed-ever.

3. Megan Thielking, "10 Million Wisdom Teeth Are Removed Each Year: That Might Be Too Many," *Vox*, last updated February 4, 2015, https://www.vox.com/2015/1/13/7539983/wisdom-teeth-necessary.

4. S. Genest-Beucher et al., "Does Mandibular Third Molar Have an Impact on Mandibular Anterior Crowding? A Literature Review," *Journal of Stomatology, Oral and Maxillofacial Surgery* 119, no. 3 (June 2018): 204–207, https://pubmed.ncbi.nlm.nih.gov/29571816/.

5. Melissa Busch, "Surgery-Free Way to Remove 3rd Molars May Be Coming," DrBiscuspid.com, June 14, 2022, https://www.drbicuspid.com/index.aspx?sec=sup&sub=cad&pag=dis&ItemID=331640.

6. US Food and Drug Administration, "Dental Amalgam Fillings," February 18, 2021, https://www.fda.gov/medical-devices/dental-devices/dental-amalgam-fillings#.

CHAPTER 9

1. Yu Zhang and J. Robert Kelly, "Dental Ceramics for Restoration and Metal-Veneering," *Dental Clinics of North America* 61, no. 4 (October 2017): 797–819, https://www.ncbi.nlm.nih.gov/pmc/articles/PMC5657342/.

2. Zhang and Kelly, "Dental Ceramics for Restoration and Metal-Veneering."

3. Mostafa Aboushahba, Hesham Katamish, and Mona Elagroudy, "Evaluation of Hardness and Wear of Surface Treated Zirconia on Enamel Wear:

An In-Vitro Study," *Future Dental Journal* 4, no. 1 (June 2018): 76–83, https://www.sciencedirect.com/science/article/pii/S2314718017300423.

4. Macrotrends, "Gold Prices—100 Year Historical Chart," accessed June 24, 2022, https://www.macrotrends.net/1333/historical-gold-prices-100-year -chart.

5. Zhang and Kelly, "Dental Ceramics for Restoration and Metal-Veneering."

CHAPTER 10

1. *Healthline*, "Root Canals and Cancer," March 14, 2019, https://www .healthline.com/health/root-canal-and-cancer.

2. Ranya Faraj Elemam and Iain Pretty, "Comparison of Success Rate of Endodontic Treatment and Implant Treatment," *ISRN (International Scholarly Research Network) Dentistry* (2011): 640509, https://www.ncbi.nlm.nih .gov/pmc/articles/PMC3168915/.

3. Centers for Disease Control and Prevention, "Tooth Loss," last reviewed January 4, 2021, accessed June 2022, https://www.cdc.gov/oralhealth/ fast-facts/tooth-loss/.

4. Centers for Disease Control and Prevention, "Periodontal Disease," last reviewed July 10, 2013, accessed June 2022, https://www.cdc.gov/oral health/conditions/periodontal-disease.htm.

5. Hannah Welk, "Periodontal Disease Costs U.S. $154B in 2018," Dr-Bicuspid.com, June 10, 2021, https://www.drbicuspid.com/index.aspx?sec=su p&sub=hyg&pag=dis&ItemID=328719.

6. American Academy of Periodontology, "New Study Links Periodontitis and COVID-19 Complications," press release, February 3, 2021, https://www.perio.org/press-release/new-study-links-periodontitis-and -covid%E2%80%9019-complications/.

7. American Academy of Periodontology, "Gum Disease and Men," accessed June 28, 2022, https://www.perio.org/for-patients/gum-disease -information/gum-disease-and-men/

8. American Academy of Periodontology, "Gum Disease and Men," accessed June 28, 2022, https://www.perio.org/for-patients/gum-disease -information/gum-disease-and-other-diseases/.

9. National Library of Medicine, "What Is an Inflammation?" November 23, 2010, last updated February 22, 2018, https://www.ncbi.nlm.nih.gov /books/NBK279298/.

10. *Healthline*, "What to Know about Periodontal Pockets," November 15, 2017, https://www.healthline.com/health/periodontal-pockets#diagnosis.

11. M. Galvan et al., "Periodontal Effects of 0.25% Sodium Hypochlorite Twice-Weekly Oral Rinse," *Journal of Periodontal Research* 49, no. 6 (December 2014): 696–702, https://pubmed.ncbi.nlm.nih.gov/24329929/.

12. Imahn Moin, "Mouth Rinsing with Bleach: A Promising Alternative to Chlorhexidine?" *Spear Education*, November 1, 2017, https://www.speared ucation.com/spear-review/2017/10/mouthrinsing-with-bleach-a-promising -alternative-to-chlorhexidine.

CHAPTER II

1. Marko Vujicic, "Dental Market Outlook: Data-Driven Insights," Health Policy Institute/American Dental Association (2019): 1–36.

2. Sonal Raikar et al., "Factors Affecting the Survival Rate of Dental Implants: A Retrospective Study," *Journal of International Society of Preventive & Community Dentistry* 7, no. 6 (November–December 2017): 351–55, https://www.ncbi.nlm.nih.gov/pmc/articles/PMC5774056/.

3. Jayachandran Prathapachandran and Neethu Suresh, "Management of Peri-implantitis," *Dental Research Journal* 9, no. 5 (September–October 2012): 516–21, https://www.ncbi.nlm.nih.gov/pmc/articles/PMC3612185/.

CHAPTER 12

1. Administration for Community Living, US Department of Health and Human Services, *2019 Profile of Older Americans*, May 2020, https://acl.gov /sites/default/files/Aging%20and%20Disability%20in%20America/2019Profil eOlderAmericans508.pdf.

2. Centers for Disease Control and Prevention, "Edentulism and Tooth Retention," last reviewed December 9, 2021, accessed September 20, 2022, https://www.cdc.gov/oralhealth/publications/OHSR-2019-edentulism-tooth -retention.html.

3. Georgetown University Health Policy Institute, "Prescription Drugs," accessed July 11, 2022, https://hpi.georgetown.edu/rxdrugs/#:~:text=More%20 than%20131%20million%20people,United%20States%20%E2%80%94%20 use%20prescription%20drugs.

4. American Dental Association, "Breastfeeding: 6 Things Nursing Moms Should Know About Dental Health," accessed July 11, 2022, https://www. mouthhealthy.org/en/az-topics/b/breastfeeding.

5. National Institute of Dental and Craniofacial Research, "The Story of Fluoridation," accessed June 15, 2022, https://www.nidcr.nih.gov/health-info /fluoride/the-story-of-fluoridation.

6. Centers for Disease Control and Prevention, "Water Fluoridation Basics," last reviewed October 1, 2021, accessed September 20, 2022, https:// www.cdc.gov/fluoridation/basics/index.htm.

7. Centers for Disease Control and Prevention, "Water Fluoridation Basics."

8. Eric Suni, "Snoring in Children," Sleep Foundation, last updated March 11, 2022, https://www.sleepfoundation.org/snoring/snoring-children.

9. Foundation for Airway Health, "Finding Connor Deegan," YouTube video, uploaded November 28, 2019, https://www.youtube.com /watch?v=QcfyPT0MQCU.

10. National Cancer Institute, "HPV and Cancer," last updated October 25, 2021, accessed September 20, 2022, https://www.cancer.gov/about -cancer/causes-prevention/risk/infectious-agents/hpv-and-cancer#:~:text=In% 20the%20United%20States%2C%20high,for%20Disease%20Control%20 (CDC).

CHAPTER 13

1. American Dental Association, "The Dentist Workforce," accessed July 15, 2022, https://www.ada.org/resources/research/health-policy-institute /dentist-workforce.

2. Bradley Munson et al., "How Did the COVID-19 Pandemic Affect Dentist Earnings?" American Dental Association Health Policy Institute Research Brief, September 2021, https://www.ada.org/-/media/project /ada-organization/ada/ada-org/files/resources/research/hpi/hpibrief_0921_1 .pdf?utm_medium=NDN.

3. Centers for Disease Control and Prevention, "States with a Dental Director," 2018, accessed September 17, 2022, https://chronicdata.cdc.gov /Oral-Health/States-with-a-Dental-Director/qek2-iyap.

CHAPTER 14

1. Peter S. Ungar, "Why We Have So Many Problems with Our Teeth," *Scientific American*, April 1, 2020, https://www.scientificamerican.com /article/why-we-have-so-many-problems-with-our-teeth/.

2. Sandra Kahn and Paul R. Ehrlich, "Why Cavemen Needed No Braces," *Stanford University Press Blog*, May 1, 2018, https://stanfordpress.typepad.com/blog/2018/05/why-cavemen-needed-no-braces.html.

3. Douglas Benn and Peter S. Vig DDS, "Estimation of X-ray Radiation Related Cancers in US Dental Offices: Is It Worth the Risk?" *Oral Surgery, Oral Medicine, Oral Pathology and Oral Radiology* 132, no. 5 (November 2021), https://www.sciencedirect.com/science/article/pii/S2212440321000742.

4. Mohamed Atfy Abd Elmotaleb et al., "Effectiveness of Using a Vibrating Device in Accelerating Orthodontic Tooth Movement: A Systemic Review and Meta-Analysis," *Journal of International Society of Preventive & Community Dentistry* 9, no. 1 (January–February 2019): 5–12, https://www.ncbi.nlm.nih.gov/pmc/articles/PMC6402256/#:~:text=Conclusion%3A,acceleration%20of%20orthodontic%20tooth%20movement.

5. Pocket Dentistry, "History, Present and Future of Aligners," accessed July 25, 2022, https://pocketdentistry.com/history-present-and-future-of-aligners/.

6. Betul Yuzbasioglu Ertugrul and Ilknur Veli, "Evaluating the Effects of Orthodontic Treatment with Clear Aligners and Conventional Brackets on Mandibular Condyle Bone Quality Using Fractal Dimension Analysis of Panoramic Radiographs," *Journal of Stomatology, Oral and Maxillofacial Surgery* 123, no. 5 (October 2022): 538–45, https://www.sciencedirect.com/science/article/abs/pii/S2468785522001616?via%3Dihub.

7. Man Hung et al., "Examination of Orthodontic Expenditures and Trends in the United States from 1996 to 2016: Disparities across Demographics and Insurance Payers," *BMC Oral Health* 21, no. 268 (May 17, 2021), https://bmcoralhealth.biomedcentral.com/articles/10.1186/s12903-021-01629-6.

8. T. F. Foley and A. H. Mamandras, "Facial Growth in Females 14 to 20 Years of Age," *American Journal of Orthodontics and Dentofacial Orthopedics* 101, no. 3 (March 1992): 248–54, https://pubmed.ncbi.nlm.nih.gov/1539552/.

9. R. J. Love, J. M. Murray, and A. H. Mamandras, "Facial Growth in Males 16 to 20 Years of Age," *American Journal of Orthodontics and Dentofacial Orthopedics* 97, no. 3 (March 1990): 200–206, https://pubmed.ncbi.nlm.nih.gov/2309666/.

10. Fernanda Angelieri et al., "Midpalatal Suture Maturation: Classification Method for Individual Assessment before Rapid Maxillary Expansion," *American Journal of Orthodontics and Dentofacial Orthopedics* 144, no. 5 (November 1, 2013), https://www.ajodo.org/article/S0889-5406(13)00746-4/fulltext.

11. David Sedaris, *Happy-Go-Lucky* (New York: Little, Brown and Company, 2022), 398.

CHAPTER 15

1. American Academy of Sleep Medicine, "Risk of Motor Vehicle Accidents Is Higher in People with Sleep Apnea," press release, March 10, 2015, https://aasm.org/risk-of-motor-vehicle-accidents-is-higher-in-people-with-sleep-apnea/.

2. Abd A. Tahrani, "Ethnic Differences in the Pathogenesis of Obstructive Sleep Apnea: Exploring Non-anatomical Factors," *Respirology* (April 17, 2017), https://onlinelibrary.wiley.com/doi/10.1111/resp.13057.

3. American Cancer Society, "Key Statistics for Oral Cavity and Oropharyngeal Cancers," last revised January 12, 2022, accessed September 17, 2022, https://cancer.org/cancer/oral-cavity-and-oropharyngeal-cancer/about/key-statistics.html.

4. Claudio Pelucchi, "Cancer Risk Associated with Alcohol and Tobacco Use: Focus on Upper Aero-digestive Tract and Liver," *Alcohol Research and Health* 29, no. 3 (2006): 193–98, https://www.ncbi.nlm.nih.gov/pmc/articles/PMC6527045/.

5. Rana Ataran et al., "The Role of Botulinum Toxin A in Treatment of Temporomandibular Joint Disorders: A Review," *Journal of Dentistry* 18, no. 3 (September 2017): 157–64, https://www.ncbi.nlm.nih.gov/pmc/articles/PMC5634354/.

6. Safe Horizon, "Human Trafficking Statistics and Facts," accessed August 5, 2022, https://www.safehorizon.org/get-informed/human-trafficking-statistics-facts/#description/.

7. US Department of State, "About Human Trafficking," accessed August 5, 2022, https://www.state.gov/humantrafficking-about-human-trafficking/.

CHAPTER 16

1. Dental AI Council, accessed January 15, 2023, https://www.dentalcouncil.org/mission.

2. US Food and Drug Administration, "Artificial Intelligence and Machine Learning in Software as a Medical Device," accessed August 30, 2022, https://www.fda.gov/medical-devices/software-medical-device-samd/artificial-intelligence-and-machine-learning-software-medical-device.

3. Thomas T. Nguyen et al., "Use of Artificial Intelligence in Dentistry: Current Clinical Trends and Research Advances," *Journal of the Canadian Dental Association* 87 (2021): 17, https://jcda.ca/l7.

4. Naseer Ahmed et al., "Artificial Intelligence Techniques: Analysis, Application, and Outcome in Dentistry—A Systematic Review," *BioMed Research International* (2021): 9751564, https://www.ncbi.nlm.nih.gov/pmc/articles/PMC8245240.

5. Nam Nguyen, Andrew H. Jheon, and Michael S. Reddy, "Embracing Precision and Data Science in Dentistry," *California Dental Association Journal* 50, no. 8 (August 2022), https://issuu.com/cdapublications/docs/cda_august_2022_issuu.

6. Divya Tandon and Joytika Rajawat, "Present and Future of Artificial Intelligence in Dentistry," *Journal of Oral Biology and Craniofacial Research* 10, no. 4 (October–December 2020): 391–96, https://www.ncbi.nlm.nih.gov/pmc/articles/PMC7394756/.

7. Netherlands Cancer Institute, "First Successful Operation with Custom 3D-Printed Titanium Lower Jaw," *Newswise*, August 4, 2022, https://www.newswise.com/articles/first-successful-operation-with-custom-3d-printed-titanium-lower-jaw?sc=dwhr&xy=10015810.

8. Nguyen et al., "Embracing Precision and Data Science in Dentistry."

9. Nguyen et al., "Embracing Precision and Data Science in Dentistry."

10. Hamin Shin et al., "Surface Activity—Tuned Metal Oxide Chemiresistor: Toward Direct and Quantitative Halitosis Diagnosis," *ACS Nano* 15, no. 9 (2021): 14207–17, https://pubs.acs.org/doi/10.1021/acsnano.1c01350.

11. Tracey Regan, "NJIT-Led Team Revitalizes Teeth through Tissue Regeneration," New Jersey Institute of Technology, June 7, 2022, https://news.njit.edu/njit-led-team-revitalizes-teeth-through-tissue-regeneration.

12. Graycen Wheeler, "Novel Material Mimics Enamel's Complex Structure with Stronger Components," *Science*, February 3, 2022, https://www.science.org/content/article/new-artificial-enamel-harder-and-more-durable-real-thing.

13. University of Washington School of Dentistry, "Trials Begin on Lozenge That Rebuilds Tooth Enamel," March 1, 2021, https://dental.washington.edu/trials-begin-on-lozenge-that-rebuilds-tooth-enamel/.

14. Theresa Pablos, "Meet Robin, the Robot in the Treatment Room," DrBicuspid.com, March 19, 2021, https://www.drbicuspid.com/index.aspx?sec=vendor&sub=webinars&pag=dis&ItemID=328209.

15. Paras Ahmad et al., "Dental Robotics: A Disruptive Technology," *Sensors* 21, no. 10 (May 2021): 33–38, https://www.ncbi.nlm.nih.gov/pmc/articles/PMC8151353/.

GLOSSARY

avulsed: knocked out; usually refers to a tooth knocked out of its socket

bitewing X-ray: an X-ray of a back tooth (or teeth) that shows the top portion of the tooth not covered by the gums (crown portion); used primarily to check for cavities

cementum: the outermost layer of the root of the tooth

crepitus: a crackling, grating sensation or sound in a joint often found in arthritis

crown: 1. the top portion of the tooth visible above the gumline; 2. a dental restoration that covers the entire tooth

dentin: the layer beneath the enamel in a tooth

edentulous: having no teeth

enamel: the outermost layer of the crown of a tooth

enameloplasty: selective drilling of enamel to reshape the contour of a tooth

endodontist: a dental specialist who does root canals and other procedures associated with the dental pulp

endosseous: within the bone

full-mouth X-ray series: a set of eighteen X-rays—fourteen periapicals and four bitewings—to evaluate the teeth, jaws, and surrounding structures

gingivitis: the earliest, reversible stage of gum disease characterized by red, puffy, bleeding gums

halitosis: bad breath

malocclusion: a bad bite characterized by upper and lower teeth that do not meet together in a stable fashion

mandible: the lower jaw

maxilla: the upper jaw

mucositis: irritation or swelling of the gum around an implant

nociceptors: sensory receptors that detect pain or nerve fibers

occlusal X-ray: an X-ray showing the chewing surfaces of teeth

occlusion: the bite

onlay: a restoration similar to a crown that covers a portion of the tooth rather than the entire tooth

osteonecrosis: spontaneous destruction of bone linked to an inadequate blood supply

osteoradionecrosis: osteonecrosis caused by radiation therapy

periapical X-ray: an X-ray of the entire tooth, including the root and the surrounding bone; used to check the overall health of the tooth, the shape of the roots, and the anatomy of the root canal system

peri-implantitis: a gum infection around an implant

periodontal disease: inflammatory disease of the tissues around the teeth; includes gingivitis and periodontitis

periodontist: a specialist who treats the supporting structures of the teeth (the gums); also place implants and extract the occasional tooth

periodontitis: the irreversible form of gum disease marked by bone loss, bleeding, inflammation, and mobility of the tooth and surrounding gums

plaque: the sticky whitish/yellowish substance containing mostly bacteria that forms around teeth

prophylaxis: a preventive treatment against disease; in the case of your teeth, a simple dental cleaning

pulp: the innermost portion of a tooth containing the nerve, blood vessels, and connective tissue

pulpotomy: removal of the top portion of the pulp

resorption: the internal or external deterioration of the root

stayplate: a temporary partial denture

subgingival: below the gumline

supraeruption: growth of a tooth beyond the imaginary plane separating upper and lower teeth

supragingival: above the gumline

tartar: calculus or hardened plaque

temporomandibular joints: the two joints connecting the lower jaw to the skull

trephination: a procedure to remove a broken implant; involves removing a core of healthy bone around the implant

xerostomia: dry mouth marked by reduced saliva flow

BIBLIOGRAPHY

Aboushahba, Mostafa, Hesham Katamish, and Mona Elagroudy. "Evaluation of Hardness and Wear of Surface Treated Zirconia on Enamel Wear: An In-Vitro Study." *Future Dental Journal* 4, no. 1 (June 2018): 76–83. https://www.sciencedirect.com/science/article/pii/S2314718017300423.

Administration for Community Living, US Department of Health and Human Services. *2019 Profile of Older Americans*. May 2020. https://acl.gov/sites/default/files/Aging%20and%20Disability%20in%20America/2019ProfileOlderAmericans508.pdf.

Ahmad, Paras, et al. "Dental Robotics: A Disruptive Technology." *Sensors* 21, no. 10 (May 2021): 3308. https://www.ncbi.nlm.nih.gov/pmc/articles/PMC8151353/.

Ahmed, Naseer, et al. "Artificial Intelligence Techniques: Analysis, Application, and Outcome in Dentistry—A Systematic Review." *BioMed Research International* (2021): 9751564. https://www.ncbi.nlm.nih.gov/pmc/articles/PMC8245240/.

Ali, Shirin. "Survey Finds More Than Half of Americans Can't Afford a $1,000 Emergency." *The Hill*, January 19, 2022. https://thehill.com/changing-america/respect/poverty/590453-survey-finds-over-half-of-americans-cant-afford-a-1000/.

American Academy of Periodontology. "Gum Disease and Men." Accessed June 28, 2022. https://www.perio.org/for-patients/gum-disease-information/gum-disease-and-men/.

———. "Gum Disease and Women." Accessed June 28, 2022. https://www.perio.org/gum-disease-information/gum-disease-and-women/.

———. "New Study Links Periodontitis and COVID-19 Complications." Press release, February 3, 2021. https://www.perio.org/press-release/new-study-links-periodontitis-and-covid%E2%80%9019-complications/.

———. "New Study Suggests the Ideal Sequence for Removing Plaque." Press release, August 29, 2018. https://www.perio.org/press-release/new-study-suggests-the-ideal-sequence-for-removing-plaque/.

American Academy of Sleep Medicine. "Risk of Motor Vehicle Accidents Is Higher in People with Sleep Apnea." Press release, March 10, 2015. https://aasm.org/risk-of-motor-vehicle-accidents-is-higher-in-people-with-sleep-apnea/.

American Association of Physicists in Medicine. "AAPM Position Statement on the Use of Patient Gonadal and Fetal Shielding." April 2, 2019. https://www.aapm.org/org/policies/details.asp?type=PP&id=2552.

American Cancer Society. "Key Statistics for Oral Cavity and Oropharyngeal Cancers." Last revised January 12, 2022. Accessed September 17, 2022. https://cancer.org/cancer/oral-cavity-and-oropharyngeal-cancer/about/key-statistics.html.

———. "Risk Factors for Oral Cavity and Oropharyngeal Cancers." Accessed June 15, 2022. https://www.cancer.org/cancer/oral-cavity-and-oropharyngeal-cancer/causes-risks-prevention/risk-factors.html.

American College of Periodontology. "New Study Suggests the Ideal Sequence for Removing Plaque." Press release, August 29, 2018. https://www.perio.org/press-release/new-study-suggests-the-ideal-sequence-for-removing-plaque/.

American College of Prosthodontists. "Facts and Figures." Accessed June 13, 2022. https://www.gotoapro.org/facts-figures/.

American Dental Association. "About Give Kids A Smile." Accessed June 14, 2022. https://www.ada.org/resources/community-initiatives/give-kids-a-smile/about-give-kids-a-smile.

———. "About the ADA." Accessed June 12, 2022. https://www.ada.org/about.

———. "American Dental Association Statement on Regular Dental Visits." *Dental Tribune*, June 13, 2013. https://us.dental-tribune.com/news/ada-issues-statement-on-regular-dental-visits/.

———. "Breastfeeding: 6 Things Nursing Moms Should Know about Dental Health." Accessed July 11, 2022. https://www.mouthhealthy.org/en/az-topics/b/breastfeeding.

————. *Dental Radiographic Examinations: Recommendations for Patient Selection and Limiting Radiation Exposure.* Last revised 2012. https://www.ada.org/-/media/project/ada-organization/ada/ada-org/files/resources/research/oral-health-topics/dental_radiographic_examinations_2012.pdf.

————. "The Dentist Workforce." Accessed July 15, 2022. https://www.ada.org/resources/research/health-policy-institute/dentist-workforce.

————. "How Many Dentists Are in Solo Practice?" Accessed June 13, 2022. https://www.ada.org/-/media/project/ada-organization/ada/ada-org/files/resources/research/hpi/hpigraphic_0121_1.pdf.

————. "Tuition, Admission, and Attrition Reports." Accessed June 13, 2022. https://www.ada.org/resources/research/health-policy-institute/dental-education.

Angelieri, Fernanda, et al. "Midpalatal Suture Maturation: Classification Method for Individual Assessment before Rapid Maxillary Expansion." *American Journal of Orthodontics and Dentofacial Orthopedics* 144, no. 5 (November 1, 2013). https://www.ajodo.org/article/S0889-5406(13)00746-4/fulltext.

Ataran, Rana, et al. "The Role of Botulinum Toxin A in Treatment of Temporomandibular Joint Disorders: A Review." *Journal of Dentistry* 18, no. 3 (September 2017): 157–64. https://ncbi.nlm.nih.gov/pmc/articles/PMC5634354/.

Beaton, Laura, Ruth Freeman, and Gerry Humphris. "Why Are People Afraid of the Dentist? Observations and Explanations." *Medical Principles and Practice* 23 (2014): 295–301.

Benn, Douglas K., and Peter S. Vig. "Estimation of X-ray Radiation Related Cancers in US Dental Offices: Is It Worth the Risk?" *Oral Surgery, Oral Medicine, Oral Pathology, and Oral Radiology* 132, no. 5 (November 2021). https://www.sciencedirect.com/science/article/pii/S2212440321000742.

Berkhout, W. E. R., G. C. H. Sanderink, and P. F. Van der Stelt. "Does Digital Radiography Increase the Number of Intraoral Radiographs?" *Dentomaxillofacial Radiology* 32, no. 2 (January 28, 2014). https://doi.org/10.1259/dmfr/97410196.

Blackwell, Debra L., Mario A. Villaroel, and Tina Norris. *Regional Variation in Private Dental Coverage and Care among Dentate Adults Aged 18–64 in the United States, 2014–2017.* NCHS Data Brief, no. 336. Hyattsville, MD: National Center for Health Statistics, 2019. https://www.cdc.gov/nchs/data/databriefs/db336-h.pdf.

Busch, Melissa. "Catalanotto: Dental Therapy Is Key to Oral Health Equity." DrBicuspid.com, June 25, 2021. https://www.drbicuspid.com/index.aspx?sec=sup&sub=hyg&pag=dis&ItemID=328821.

―――. "Surgery-Free Way to Remove 3rd Molars May Be Coming." DrBicuspid.com, June 14, 2022. https://www.drbicuspid.com/index.aspx?sec=s up&sub=cad&pag=dis&ItemID=331640.

Centers for Disease Control and Prevention. "Edentulism and Tooth Retention." Last reviewed December 9, 2021. Accessed September 20, 2022. https://www.cdc.gov/oralhealth/publications/OHSR-2019-edentulism -tooth-retention.html.

―――. "The Electromagnetic Spectrum: Ionizing Radiation." Last reviewed June 29, 2021. Accessed June 29, 2021. https://www.cdc.gov/nceh/radia tion/ionizing_radiation.html.

―――. "It's All about the Energy—Measuring Radiation." Last reviewed December 7, 2015. Accessed June 29, 2021. https://www.cdc.gov/nceh /radiation/energy.html#dose.

―――. "Periodontal Disease." Last reviewed July 10, 2013. Accessed June 2022. https://www.cdc.gov/oralhealth/conditions/periodontal-disease.html.

―――. "States with a Dental Director." 2018. Accessed September 17, 2022. https://chronicdata.cdc.gov/Oral-Health/States-with-a-Dental -Director/qek2-iyap.

―――. "Tooth Loss." Last reviewed January 4, 2021. Accessed June 2022. https://www.cdc.gov/oralhealth/fast-facts/tooth-loss/.

―――. "Water Fluoridation Basics." Last reviewed October 1, 2021. Accessed September 20, 2022. https://www.cdc.gov/fluoridation/basics/index. htm.

Datta, Yogita. "The U.S. Toothpaste Market: A Competitive Profile." *Journal of Economics and Public Finance* 6, no. 1 (February 27, 2020): 145–67. https://www.researchgate.net/publication/339538350_The_US_Tooth paste_Market_A_Competitive_Profile.

Dental AI Council. Accessed January 15, 2023, https://www.dentalaicouncil .org/mission.

Domino, Donna. "Calif. Dentist to Pay $80,000 in Yelp Case." DrBicuspid. com, May 17, 2011. https://www.drbicuspid.com/index.aspx?sec=nws&sub =rad&pag=dis&ItemID=307681.

Edwards, Tony. "U.S. Dental Spending Projected to Reach 203B by 2027." DrBicuspid.com, June 7, 2021. https://www.drbicuspid.com/index.aspx?se c=sup&sub=pmt&pag=dis&ItemID=324228.

EINPresswire. "Cosmetic Dentistry Market Size to Worth USD 35.66 Billion in 2028." Press release, June 22, 2022. https://www.einnews.com /pr_news/577915674/cosmetic-dentistry-market-size-to-worth-usd-35-66 -billion-in-2028-at-a-cagr-of-6-3-says-reports-and-data.

Elemam, Ranya Faraj, and Iain Pretty. "Comparison of the Success Rate of Endodontic Treatment and Implant Treatment." *ISRN (International Scholarly Research Network) Dentistry* (2011): 640509. https://www.ncbi.nlm.nih.gov/pmc/articles/PMC3168915/.

Elmotaleb, Mohamed Atfy Abd, et al. "Effectiveness of Using a Vibrating Device in Acclerating Orthodontic Tooth Movement: A Systematic Review and Meta-Analysis." *Journal of International Society of Preventive & Community Dentistry* 9, no. 1 (January–February 2019): 5–12. https://www.ncbi.nlm.nih.gov/pmc/articles/PMC6402256/.

Ertugrul, Betol Yuzbasioglu, and Ilknur Veli. "Evaluating the Effects of Orthodontic Treatment with Clear Aligners and Conventional Brackets on Mandibular Condyle Bone Quality Using Fractal Dimension Analysis of Panoramic Radiographs." *Journal of Stomatology, Oral and Maxillofacial Surgery* 123, no. 5 (October 2022): 538–45. https://www.sciencedirect.com/science/article/abs/pii/S2468785522001616?via%3Dihub.

European Commission. "Radiation Protection." Last modified 2014. https://energy.ec.europa.eu/system/files/2014-11/156_0.pdf.

Feliz-Matos, Leandro, Luis Miguel Hernandez, and Ninoska Abreu. "Dental Bleaching Techniques; Hydrogen-Carbamide Peroxides and Light Sources for Activation, an Update." *Open Dentistry Journal* 8 (2014): 264–68. https://www.ncbi.nlm.nih.gov/pmc/articles/PMC4311381/.

Foley, T. F., and A. H. Mamandras. "Facial Growth in Females 14 to 20 Years of Age." *American Journal of Orthodontics and Dentofacial Orthopedics* 101, no. 3 (March 1992): 248–54. https://pubmed.ncbi.nlm.nih.gov/1539552/.

Fortune Business Insights. "Dental CAD/CAM Market Size, Share and Covid-19 Impact Analysis." March 2022. Accessed June 24, 2022. https://www.fortunebusinessinsights.com/dental-cad-cam-market-105080.

———. "Medical Tourism Market." February 2022. Accessed June 14, 2022. https://www.fortunebusinessinsights.com/industry-reports/medical-tourism-market-100681.

Foundation for Airway Health. "Finding Connor Deegan." YouTube video, uploaded November 28, 2019. https://www.youtube.com/watch?v=QcfyPT0MQCU.

Galvan, M., et al. "Periodontal Effects of 0.25% Sodium Hypochlorite Twice-Weekly Oral Rinse: A Pilot Study." *Journal of Periodontology* 49, no. 6 (December 2014): 646–702. https://pubmed.ncbi.nlm.nih.gov/24329929/.

Garla, Bharath Kumar, G. Satish, and D. T. Divya. "Dental Insurance: A Systematic Review." *Journal of International Society of Preventive & Com-*

munity Dentistry 4, suppl. 2 (December 2014): S73–S77. https://www. ncbi.nlm.nih.gov/pmc/articles/PMC4278106/.

Genest-Beucher, S., et al. "Does Mandibular Third Molar Have an Impact on Mandibular Anterior Crowding? A Literature Review." *Journal of Stomatology, Oral and Maxillofacial Surgery* 119, no. 3 (June 2018): 204–207. https://www.pubmed.ncbi.nlm.nih.gov/29571816/.

Georgetown University Health Policy Institute. "Prescription Drugs." Accessed July 11, 2022. https://hpi.georgetown.edu/rxdrugs/#:~:text=More%20 than%20131%20million%20people,United%20States%20 %E2%80%94%20use%20prescription%20drugs.

Giannobile, W. V., et al. "Patient Stratification for Preventive Care in Dentistry." *Journal of Dental Research* 92, no. 8 (August 2013): 694–701.

Gupta, Sanjay. *Keep Sharp: Build a Better Brain at Any Age.* New York: Simon & Schuster. 2021.

Healthline. "Root Canals and Cancer." March 14, 2019. https://www.health line.com/health/root-canal-and-cancer.

———. "What to Know about Periodontal Pockets." November 15, 2017. https://www.healthline.com/health/dental-oral-health-receding-gums#prevention.

Hung, Man, et al. "Examination of Orthodontic Expenditures and Trends in the United States from 1996 to 2013: Disparities across Demographics and Insurance Payers." *BMC Oral Health* 21, no. 268 (May 17, 2021). https:// bmcoralhealth.biomedcentral.com/articles/10.1186/s12903-021-01629-6.

Kahn, Sandra, and Paul R. Ehrlich. "Why Cavemen Needed No Braces." *Stanford University Press Blog,* May 1, 2018. https://stanfordpress.type pad.com/blog/2018/05/why-cavemen-needed-no-braces.html.

Love, R. J., J. M. Murray, and A. H. Mamandras. "Facial Growth in Males 16 to 20 Years of Age." *American Journal of Orthodontics and Dentofacial Orthopedics* 97, no. 3 (March 1990): 200–206. https://pubmed.ncbi.nlm. nih.gov/2309666/.

MacDonald, Fiona. "Evidence Is Mounting That Routine Wisdom Teeth Removal Is a Waste of Time." *Science Alert,* October 28, 2016. https:// www.sciencealert.com/no-you-probably-don-t-need-to-get-your-wisdom-teeth-removed-ever.

Macrotrends. "Gold Prices—100 Year Historical Chart." Accessed June 24, 2022. https://www.macrotrends.net/1333/historical-gold-prices-100-year -chart.

Moin, Imahn. "Mouth Rinsing with Bleach: A Promising Alternative to Chlorhexidine?" *Spear Education,* November 1, 2017. https://www.

speareducation.com/spear-review/2017/10/mouthrinsing-with-bleach-a
-promising-alternative-to-chlorhexidine.

Munson, Bradley, et al. "How Did the COVID-19 Pandemic Affect Dentist
Earnings?" American Dental Association Health Policy Institute Research
Brief, September 2021. https://www.ada.org/-/media/project/ada-organi
zation/ada/ada-org/files/resources/research/hpi/hpibrief_0921_1.pdf?utm
_medium=NDN.

Naidu, Arti S., et al. "Over-the-Counter Tooth Whitening Agents: A Review
of Literature." *Brazilian Dental Journal* 31, no. 3 (May–June 2020). https://
www.scielo.br/j/bdj/a/yjx5CcCCQzRWqhzFKVSgVVK/?lang=en.

National Cancer Institute. "HPV and Cancer." Last updated October 25,
2021. Accessed September 20, 2022. https://www.cancer.gov/about-cancer
/causes-prevention/risk/infectious-agents/hpv-and-cancer#:~:text=In%20
the%20United%20States%2C%20high,for%20Disease%20Control%20
(CDC).

National Institute of Dental and Craniofacial Research. "The Story of Fluoridation." Accessed June 15, 2022. https://www.nidcr.nih.gov/health-info/
fluoride/the-story-of-fluoridation.

National Library of Medicine. "What Is an Inflammation?" November 23,
2010. Last updated February 22, 2018. https://www.ncbi.nlm.nih.gov
/books/NBK279298/.

Netherlands Cancer Institute. "First Successful Operation with Custom 3D-
Printed Titanium Lower Jaw." *Newswise*, August 4, 2022. https://www.
newswise.com/articles/first-successful-operation-with-custom-3d-printed
-titanium-lower-jaw?sc=dwhr&xy=10015810.

Nguyen, Nam, Andrew H. Jheon, and Michael S. Reddy. "Embracing Precision and Data Science in Dentistry." *California Dental Association Journal*
50, no. 8 (August 2022): 441–52. https://issuu.com/cdapublications/docs
/cda_august_2022_issuu.

Nguyen, Thomas T., et al. "Use of Artificial Intelligence in Dentistry: Current Clinical Trends and Research Advances." *Journal of the Canadian
Dental Association* 87 (2021): l7. https://jcda.ca/l7.

Omicron Kappa Upsilon Bylaws. Last revised March 8, 2015. https://okusu
preme.org/about-oku/bylaws.

Owens, Pamela L., Richard J. Manski, and Audrey J. Weiss. "Emergency Department Visits Involving Dental Conditions 2018." *Agency for Healthcare
Research and Quality* (August 2021): 1–18. https://www.hcup-us.ahrq.gov
/reports/statbriefs/sb280-Dental-ED-Visits-2018.pdf.

Pablos, Theresa. "Meet Robin, the Robot in the Treatment Room." DrBi-cuspid.com, March 19, 2021. https://www.drbicuspid.com/index.aspx?sec=vendor&sub=webinars&pag=dis&ItemID=328209.

Pauwels, Ruben. "History of Dental Radiography: Evolution of 2D and 3D Imaging Modalities." *Medical Physics International Journal* (April 2020): 235–77. https://www.researchgate.net/publication/340444478_HISTORY_OF_DENTAL_RADIOGRAPHY_EVOLUTION_OF_2D_AND_3D_IMAGING_MODALITIES.

Pelucchi, Claudio. "Cancer Risk Associated with Alcohol and Tobacco Use: Focus on Upper Aero-digestive Tract and Liver." *Alcohol Research and Health* 29, no. 3 (2006): 193–98. https://www.ncbi.nlm.nih.gov/pmc/articles/PMC6527045/.

Pocket Dentistry. "History, Present and Future of Aligners." Accessed July 27, 2022. https://pocketdentistry.com/history-present-and-future-of-aligners/.

Prathapachandran, Jayachandran, and Neethu Suresh. "Management of Peri-implantitis." *Dental Research Journal* 9, no. 5 (September–October 2012): 516–21. https://www.ncbi.nlm.nih.gov/pmc/articles/PMC3612185/.

Raikar, Sonal, et al. "Factors Affecting the Survival Rate of Dental Implants: A Retrospective Study." *Journal of International Society of Preventive & and Community Dentistry* 7, no. 6 (November–December 2017): 351–55. https://www.ncbi.nlm.nih.gov/pmc/articles/PMC5774056/.

Regan, Tracey. "NJIT-Led Team Revitalizes Teeth through Tissue Regeneration." New Jersey Institute of Technology. June 7, 2022. https://news.njit.edu/njit-led-team-revitalizes-teeth-through-tissue-regeneration.

Rehan, Kelly. "To DSO or Not to DSO?" *Academy of General Dentistry Journal* (September 14, 2020). https://www.agd.org/about-agd/public ations-news/newsroom/newsroom-list/2020/09/14/to-dso-or-not-to-dso.

Safe Horizon. "Human Trafficking." Accessed August 5, 2022. https://www.safehorizon.org/get-informed/human-trafficking-statistics-facts/#description/.

Saint Louis, Catherine. "Feeling Guilty about Not Flossing? Maybe There's No Need." *New York Times*, August 2, 2016. https://www.nytimes.com/2016/08/03/health/flossing-teeth-cavities.html.

Scardella, David A. "CBCT Purchasing Guide: How to Choose the Perfect Machine." *Academy of General Dentistry Newsroom*, February 17, 2020. https://www.agd.org/about-agd/publications-news/newsroom/newsroom-list/2020/02/17/cbct-purchasing-guide-how-to-choose-the-perfect-machine.

Schiff, Allen M. "Tracking Dental Practice Overhead and What the Results Mean." *Dental Economics*, March 31, 2021. https://www.dentaleconomics. com/practice/overhead-and-profitability/article/14201431/tracking-dental -practice-overhead-and-what-the-results-mean.

Sedaris, David. *Happy-Go-Lucky*. New York: Little, Brown and Company, 2022.

Shanbhag, Vagish Kumar L. "Oil Pulling for Maintaining Oral Hygiene—A Review." *Journal of Traditional and Complementary Medicine* 7, no. 1 (January 2017): 106–109. https://www.ncbi.nlm.nih.gov/pmc/articles /PMC5198813/.

Shin, Hamin, et al. "Surface Activity—Tuned Metal Oxide Chemiresistor: Toward Direct and Quantitative Halitosis Diagnosis." *ACS Nano* 15, no. 9 (2021): 14207–17. https://pubs.acs.org/doi/10.1021/acsnano.1c01350.

Smerling, Robert H. "Tossing Flossing?" *Harvard Health Blog*, August 17, 2016. https://www.health.harvard.edu/blog/tossing-flossing-2016081710196.

Solana, Kimber. "HPI: Dental Spending Decreased in 2020." *ADA News*, December 30, 2021. https://www.ada.org/publications/ada-news/2021 /december/hpi-dental-spending-decreased-in-2020.

Suni, Eric. "Snoring in Children." Sleep Foundation. Last updated March 11, 2022. https://www.sleepfoundation.org/snoring/snoring-children.

Tahrani, Abd A. "Ethnic Differences in the Pathogenesis of Obstructive Sleep Apnea: Exploring Non-anatomical Factors." *Respirology* (April 17, 2017). https://onlinelibrary.wiley.com/doi/10.1111/resp.13057.

Tandon, Divya, and Jyotika Rajawat. "Present and Future of Artificial Intelligence in Dentistry." *Journal of Oral Biology and Craniofacial Research* 10, no. 4 (October–December 2020): 391–96. https://www.ncbi.nlm.nih .gov/pmc/articles/PMC7394756/.

Thielking, Megan. "10 Million Wisdom Teeth Are Removed Each Year: That Might Be Too Many." *Vox*. Last updated February 4, 2015. https://www .vox.com/2015/1/13/7539983/wisdom-teeth-necessary.

Ungar, Peter S. "Why We Have So Many Problems with Our Teeth." *Scientific American*, April 1. 2020. https://www.scientificamerican.com/article/ why-we-have-so-many-problems-with-our-teeth/.

University of Washington School of Dentistry. "Trials Begin on Lozenge That Rebuilds Tooth Enamel." March 1, 2021. https://dental.washington.edu /trials-begin-on-lozenge-that-rebuilds-tooth-enamel/.

US Department of State. "About Human Trafficking." Accessed August 5, 2022. https://www.state.gov/humantrafficking-about-human-trafficking/.

US Food and Drug Administration. "Artificial Intelligence and Machine Learning in Software as a Medical Device." Accessed August 30, 2022.

https://www.fda.gov/medical-devices/software-medical-device-samd/
artificial-intelligence-and-machine-learning-software-medical-device.
———. "Dental Amalgam Fillings." February 18, 2021. https://www.fda.gov
/medical-devices/dental-devices/dental-amalgam-fillings#.
Vujicic, Marko. "Dental Market Outlook: Data-Driven Insights." Health
Policy Institute/American Dental Association. (2019): 1–36.
Welk, Hannah. "Periodontal Disease Cost U.S. $154B in 2018." DrBicuspid
.com, June 10, 2021. https://www.drbicuspid.com/index.aspx?sec=sup&su
b=hyg&pag=dis&ItemID=328719.
What's Cooking America. "Teeth Whitening." Accessed June 22,
2022. https://whatscookingamerica.net/healthbeauty/teethwhi
tening.htm#:~:text=According%20to%20the%20American%20
Academy,whitening%20products%20last%20year%20alone.
Wheeler, Graycen. "Novel Material Mimics Enamel's Complex Structure
with Stronger Components." *Science*, February 3, 2022. https://www
.science.org/content/article/new-artificial-enamel-harder-and-more-durable
-real-thing.
Yeginsu, Ceylan. "Why Medical Tourism Is Drawing Patients Even in a
Pandemic." *New York Times*, January 16, 2021. https://www.nytimes.
com/2021/01/19/travel/medical-tourism-coronavirus-pandemic.html.
Zhang, Yu, and J. Robert Kelly. "Dental Ceramics for Restoration and Metal
-Veneering." *Dental Clinics of North America* 61, no. 4 (October 2017):
797–819. https://www.ncbi.nlm.nih.gov/pmc/articles/PMC5657342/.

INDEX

ABOUT THE AUTHOR

Dr. Teresa Yang has practiced dentistry in the Los Angeles area for more than thirty years. She started and developed two practices from scratch, which is unique in today's insurance-driven world. Dr. Yang operates under the philosophy of putting the patient's interest first: A person is more than a mouth and a set of teeth.

With a BA with distinction from Stanford University and a DDS from UCLA, Dr. Yang graduated cum laude at the top of her dental school class. Over the years, she has taught clinical dentistry and patient management at UCLA School of Dentistry. Dr. Yang has also written extensively on dental topics. She is the editor of *WestViews*, a publication of the Western Los Angeles Dental Society.

Dr. Yang is a member of the Forbes Health Advisory Board. She is also a member of the UCLA School of Dentistry Board of Counselors. She has served as a trustee at the California Dental Association (CDA), as a member of the CDA Foundation Board, and as a past chair of the CDA Peer Review Council. Dr. Yang has lectured widely on conflict resolution and peer review.